FIGHTING FOR OUR LIVES

Kit Mouat is a cancer patient and a founder of Cancer Contact. Her previous publications include:

What Humanism Is About (1962)
Time Smoulders and other poems (1971)
Poems of an Angry Dove (1975)

All royalties from this book will go to support the work of Cancer Contact.

KIT MOUAT

FIGHTING FOR OUR LIVES

AN INTRODUCTION TO LIVING WITH CANCER

With a preface by
SHEILA HANCOCK

heretic books

First published March 1984 by Heretic Books
(GMP Publishers Ltd), P O Box 247, London N15 6RW.
Send s.a.e. for our catalogue.

British Library Cataloguing in Publication Data

Mouat, Kit
Fighting for our lives.
1. Cancer -- Treatment
I. Title
616.99'406 RC270.8

ISBN 0-946097-14-3

Cover by Louis Mackay

Photoset by Shanta Thawani, 25 Natal Road, London N11 2HU
Printed and bound by Hartnoll Printers Ltd,
Bodmin, Cornwall PL31 1EG

Preface

The orthodox medical establishment has made some progress in the battle against cancer, but not enough. There is a growing belief in the potential of alternative medicine, and a time must surely come when the medical world recognises this and works alongside these other methods towards cure or, better still, prevention.

From my own experience I know the helplessness that can engulf you when cancer is diagnosed and the difficulty in obtaining truly informed and wide-ranging advice, not to mention compassionate support. The Hospice Movement does this superbly, but it is too small as yet to cover all the people who need help.

Groups like Cancer Contact should be set up everywhere to provide the support and therapies that have been proved to help people in the life-and-death fight against cancer. This book should give inspiration for this to happen. I hope so.

Sheila Hancock

To Kathleen, whose courage we hope was infectious

I. Living With Cancer

Cancer Contact grew by chance out of the Mid-Sussex Homoeopathic Group during 1982. Talking generally about cancer, and items in the local press and on radio, brought in 11 members. There wasn't room in the sitting-room where we met for many more, and we were all women until one man joined us in the following spring. Some of us have had primary cancer and want to avoid a recurrence; others have had or still have secondaries and are even more urgently concerned with survival. We share information and problems, discuss symptoms and treatments, borrow and lend books, and find it comforting to be with others who share our experience of a life-threatening disease. The ease with which we talk to one another is in direct contrast to the frigid failures in communication most of us have suffered with a GP, surgeon or consultant. It is good to find that you are not the only one to have been made to feel guilty for wanting to be treated as an adult in a democracy, rather than as a disobedient child in a Jane Eyre orphanage! Even the hurt and despair we have suffered at the way we or our nearest and dearest have been told that we have cancer, is soothed in one another's company. Only together can we medically 'let our hair down'. Courage to beat the system (if that is the only way to beat the disease) begets courage: gratitude for the humanity and patience of all those who — in or outside the medical profession — have shown genuine concern and interest, circulates and shines like a searchlight in a dark night. Their co-operation is our life-line when our own energies flag and self-preservation seems altogether too much bother.

We have all been through the orthodox mill, with surgery, radiotherapy or chemotherapy. Some of us have had all three. We may have agreed to be operated on, irradiated or drugged, only out of fear of being labelled 'trouble makers', or of letting down our families. We are also usually given no choice and may find ourselves swept along on the hospital tide with no time or encouragement to think for ourselves, until it is all over and too late. Few of us have been given enough information about the long-term and side effects of the orthodox cancer treatments. No one tells us that there are responsible, medically qualified people practising unorthodox cancer treatments, inside and outside the National Health Service, and with good results.

When the experts have done all they can for us, we are on our own. We can go away and try to forget that we ever had cancer (not so easy if you are now minus a breast or two) and believe that we are 'cured'; but we shall, for a while anyway, be expected to have regular checks to see just how 'cured' we are. Or we can start facing up to the facts of life and death, in which cancer has for us become an integral part. Oscar Wilde wrote: 'To regret one's own experience is to arrest one's whole development. To deny one's own experience is to put a lie into the lips of one's own life.'

In our situation it is not easy to condone the indoctrinated conservatism of the medical profession. Doctors have, understandably, often been considered as gods, 'hatching and despatching' life, and there still lingers a dangerous hangover of divine paternalism. Sadly this belief in absolute truth and the resultant closed minds are also found in part of the alternative medical society, which is producing its own dogmas and myths. Old-style religion goes on about 'Sin, Hellfire and Redemption'; the New Age cancer gurus talk about 'Personality Defects' and healing by a psychological overhaul — strictly under their guidance, of course. Old and New both add guilt to the problems that already exist. A relative of a cancer patient wrote to Cancer Contact to tell us that the family had been unable to overcome their GP's refusal to provide a referral letter to the homoeopathic consultant (MB, NS, MRCP and DPM) whom the patient wanted to see. He refused this on the grounds that homoeopathy might interfere with the orthodox treatment. He clearly had no intention of trying to find out if this really was a danger, and the patient could not face the hassle of arguing with him.

It is a tragedy that orthodox and unorthodox oncologists (cancer specialists) cannot co-operate more for the sake of their patients. Until they can all put aside their prejudices, we shall continue to suffer and die unnecessarily. Of course the diagnosis of cancer, even if the prognosis is good, prompts us to re-examine our life-style. Now is the time to give up smoking, and to examine both our diet and our ability to cope with the stress that is inevitable for any thinking person in the 1980s. It is balance we want to achieve, but it must be our own balance, with no striving after some imposed or imaginary norm. Perhaps some of us get our priorities wrong, with duty and self-interest out of proportion. But, as Dr Edward Bach emphasised, what we need is to feel 'more like ourselves' — not less.

Members of Cancer Contact are as varied in personalities, backgrounds and beliefs as we are in age. We are (or were before marriage) librarian, pharmacist, nurse, insurance clerk, in advertising, bookseller, horticulturist, journalist, author, magistrate and full-time mother and home-maker. We are a good mix-up: carnivores and vegetarians, extraverts and introverts, atheists, agnostics, Christians and 'don't knows'. There are feminists and non-feminists: one woman mourns the fact that cancer has robbed her of the opportunity for more than two children of her own, another has no regrets that she and her husband agreed long ago to be childless. Few of us believe that there is a 'cancer personality', or that it would be scientifically possible to prove such a theory one way or the other. Thinking laterally, however, it might be interesting to see if there is a common personality factor among the people whom cancer patients choose to live with!

Perhaps some of us expected to find confirmation that we had all been to some extent pre-destined to get cancer because of our family history, but this was not so. Hormonal imbalance was a common suggested cause, but who knows how many cancer-free citizens are similarly affected? Did the removal of certain organs threaten the efficiency of the immune system? Maybe, but you could always find a 'terminal' cancer of some vital part of the body 'cured' by some unidentifiable stimulus to the body's defences, which shudder into action just when the last post is about to sound.

We accept that cancer is not one but hundreds of related diseases, and believe that none is likely to be cured simply by attacking local symptoms — be it with knife, rays or drugs. It is the whole person who is ill and must be treated, and that is why homeopathy is so valuable, working constitutionally as it does, seeing each patient not as a collection of unrelated symptoms but as a unique individual in whom every problem is relevant.

Dr Hans Nieper of Hanover, the eminent German oncologist, has said that there is no sharp line dividing those who have cancer from those who do not. The success of treatment is in the long term dependent upon the body's power to resist the disease wherever and whenever it appears. Many of us may have had cancer and beaten it, in the same way that some people have calcified patches on their lungs where TB came and went without causing any trouble. When secondary cancers are diagnosed without identifying the primaries, it may be because the primaries have done just this. Primary cancer, like a mild heart attack, can serve as a life-saving warning if we take enough note of it.

Until we know exactly what causes cancer cells to go berserk, we cannot condone medical closed minds and prejudices that restrict our own freedom to investigate and experiment. Still less should we smile upon the excuses of those whose vested interests would be threatened should cancer preventives and cures be found, and the 'alternative therapies prove more successful than the orthodox.

The subject of cancer research is depressing. For all the millions of pounds and dollars spent on it, very little progress has been made, indeed in some areas none at all, or the situation is even worse than it was. We read in 1980 that 'drug therapy for breast cancer has not made any significant difference to survival rates' since 1970 (*Guardian* 15th March 1980). Thirteen thousand women die of breast cancer every year. One in 17 women is affected by it, and one in 8 whose mothers had breast cancer. Someone should do some careful costing to discover how much money has been made out of the drugs given to such women. It is said that more people make money out of cancer than die from it.

Cancer research virtually ignores cancer as a constitutional disease and concentrates on animal experiments. In fact animals probably vary as much from one another as do humans, and many of the tested animals may have the vital safety factor that ensures that some living creatures never get cancer in spite of a lifetime of cancer-provoking situations. It is the questions that are being asked that are wrong; not just the answers. What we urgently need to know is what it is that the cancer-free people (and animals) have that we cancer patients lack.

It is a scandal and a tragedy that funds go so rarely into alternative methods of cancer treatment. The Imperial Cancer Research Fund states that it 'cannot research the whole, wide field of cancer'. But who decides which field is to be neglected? I received a letter recently from Canada, about a middle-aged man with 'terminal' cancer who is fighting a campaign against the restricted employment of funds. He believes that it is essential for more money to be spent on investigating alternative methods of cancer treatment. He was himself involved with the 'Marathon of Hope', in which the young athlete Terry Fox, who lost a leg from cancer, set out to run across Canada to raise money for research, but died before he had covered more than half the distance. There was a surplus of money raised, but the cancer powers-that-be refuse to authorise its being used for testing what it calls 'quack' cures. If medical treatment is labelled 'quack' when it is considered to be ineffective — and especially when a lot of money is made out of it — then most orthodox cancer treatment deserves the epithet. It is surely asking for trouble to allow cancer research to be directed by those whose fortunes depend on selling cancer drugs and technology.

No one in Cancer Contract had been given any advice from the allopaths (orthodox medicos) as to how to look after their general health and avoid a repeat breakdown. Some women who had had one or more mastectomies had not even been told how important it is to avoid injections, pressure, etc. on the arm on the operation side. Most of us also had the impression that, when it came to secondaries, the doctors had already given us up for lost and were more inhibited and afraid than we were. All they had to offer was more of the surgery, rays or drugs which had, after all, failed to prevent the spread of the disease in the first place. The doctors' attitude wasn't just that 'there is nothing more *we* can do for you' but that 'there is nothing more *to be done* that will be of the slightest use'. If we turned at this point to alternative therapies we were 'irresponsible': we might have been claiming rights over *their* bodies instead of over our own! If we then had a remission we were told 'it would have happened anyway'; no one wanted to know what we had been doing. No one even asked. We found that once we turned from the path of orthodoxy, we were at best an embarrassment to them and at worst a threat to their cherished prejudices, which they wouldn't give up over our dead bodies. It was as though we were telling them that Father Christmas didn't exist. There were exceptions, of course, as can be seen in some of these stories; but they should have been the rule. We have given our medical advisers stars. Five (as with hotels) is exceptionally good; doctors with no stars are those whom we would not wish on our enemies.

The general attitude amongst doctors and consultants to our unorthodox alternatives was that 'homoeopathy is faith healing' and its remedies 'placebos', which the patient must realise do not work! According to them, vitamins were a waste of time and money which, in the NHS, should be spent on tranquilisers, sleeping pills and painkillers. Preventive medicine was none of their business. Relaxation and meditation were harmless enough — some doctors even recommended them — but herbalism and reflexology were barely removed from witchcraft. The unspoken medical maxim 'We have made up our minds, don't confuse us with facts' was not good for our morale. It all added up to the sort of negative, pessimistic thinking which sick people should be allowed to go without. It paid no tribute to genuine scepticism, and no respect to reason, with which both orthodox and unorthodox claims need and deserve to be treated. It made a mockery of a truly scientific method of enquiry.

Diet is a subject, like sex and death, which few doctors are trained to deal with. Yet in 1979 it was reported that many cancer patients were starving for lack of the necessary nutrition in hospital wards. We were fortunate to have within reasonable distance two homoeopathic physicians especially interested in diet, although not all of us could afford their private charges.

Max Gerson, the German physician whom Albert Schweitzer considered 'a medical genius' [24]*, had long since caused amusement by using black coffee enemas as a means of ridding the body of toxins; but if you are cured of malignant melanoma (as one of our friends was) you stop laughing. None of us wanted to make life more difficult with food fads; several of us disliked cooking and meal-getting anyway,but until we were better informed we had to use ourselves as guinea-pigs and take whatever steps seemed most appropriate for our own situation, digestion and temperament. Dr Richard Mackarnass [36] had shown that some foods can cause mental as well as physical breakdowns. To leave diet out of the cancer reckoning didn't make sense.

Our doctors, however, continued to consider the tumour as the cancer; all they had to do was cut it out, burn it to death with radiation, or kill it with drugs. The rest of the body, now teeming with dead healthy cells as well as dead cancer cells, was expected to carry on regardless. We live in a society addicted to drugs, from alcohol and nicotine to Valium. It is illegal to smoke cannabis, but unpopular to question or refuse the drugs we are told to take in hospital. Out of the hundreds of millions of pounds spent on advertising drugs, 80 per cent is directed at our doctors. More than £3,000 p.a. is spent on each one of them, trying to persuade him or her to prescribe one orthodox drug rather than another. One GP described the sales representatives as 'pestilential', but in their turn the reps summed up their doctor-customers as 'Gullibles', 'Pseudo-Sophisticates', 'Motherly Types', 'Snobs' and 'Ignorants'.

Small or large bribes are taken for granted in most surgeries and chemists. Of course the doctors are only

*Numbers in square brackets refer to the list of reference books at the end of this book.

the 'middle-men'; the patients are the consumers, and the choices made from the advertising material are a matter of their life or death. Hospital wards are crowded with people suffering not from a disease but from the side effects of drugs given for a disease. It is quite possible now to be 'Cured to Death' [39]. This cannot happen with homoeopathy, which has for nearly 200 years been a major target of the pharmaceutical industry, and as a result is also the target of much opposition from doctors. If they were given only serious, unbiased reports, instead of flash commercials, we patients would not have to battle with their antagonism. We need all our energy for fighting cancer; we have none to spare. If we question what we are told to swallow in hospital or elsewhere, we should win praise, not a rebuff. Chemists who refuse to supply homoeopathic remedies on prescription must be reminded that they are duty bound to do so, according to their own professional code of ethics.

It is not only the drug pushers we have to watch: we are all media-fodder for the manufacturers of foods that everyone would be better without, from hamburgers and fizzy drinks to the sweets and carbohydrates which we did without during the war — much to our advantage.

The personal stories in this book do not pretend to tell the whole truth and nothing but — even if it were known. We did not know one another well enough to probe, say, into the effects of cancer on sexuality. If the whole person is to be considered, such questions must be of interest, and are inevitably involved with what are quoted as 'problems with relationships' and even 'job dissatisfaction' for women whose job is home-bound. It did not go without mention that the emphasis usually placed on female so-called 'promiscuity' as a cause of cervical cancer was ironic considering the failure to refer to the traditional lack of sexual hygiene in British men and boys. It is not by chance that Jewish women and nuns generally escape this particular form of the disease. There were also comments about sex-roles: 'I really resent being a woman, especially at Christmas time when everything is left to me!' said one. Another, too much of an individualist to join the group, who died after a brave but wholly orthodox battle, had written: 'I don't make friends easily, and I have always kept away from groups. Many of the things I have wished to do have had to be suppressed in the interests of being the "administrative assistant" to the one with all the creative talents! It has not always been easy for me, but when one makes that kind of choice, one has to stick to it.' But was that 'kind of choice' worse for women, or were men equally oppressed by the role thrust on them by society as 'head of the family' and traditional (if not always in fact) breadwinner-in-chief? Women with no status other than that reflected by their husbands might well be more ambitious for them than was good for either of them. Woman as 'Eve', the source of nourishment and Evil, feels guilty if she doesn't enjoy nourishing and cooking. Adam, however, is accounted innocent if he cannot stand hunting, gardening, DIY or even bank-managing. Many people are not happy with their work, and may not be successful in human relationships, but they don't all have cancer.

We did not at first discuss death, mostly (we liked to think) because we were all concentrating so much on survival that the subject seemed irrelevant. However, as our youngest member became increasingly ill and disabled, it was clear that we would have more facts to bring into focus and that we would have to learn how to talk positively with any bereaved people who wanted to join us. One cannot face one's own death without the anxiety of what such bereavement will do to our loved ones; this is perhaps the hardest problem of all. It must be possible, however (some of us felt), to strive positively and with determination for life, while at the same time accepting our own mortality. After all, any of us might be the victims of a traffic accident or some other disaster, and die while still cancer-free. It was best to make our wills while we were fit and able and, if we believed in it, to sign the declaration form for voluntary euthanasia, which might prevent our being kept alive after life had become less than human and robbed of all dignity. We knew that wanting to die did not make death any more likely, as far too many people in geriatric wards know to their cost. We did not have to fear discussion about death. Rather we might suffer from being unable to express irrational fears, denying ourselves the mutual comfort and support of the group.

There were black patches of depression for most of us from time to time, and these were not helped by reading that depression could itself lead the immune system to break down, for then the next problem was how to avoid depression about getting depressed! There had to be an exit from that one, and one of the best was visualisation therapy. The question (in the questionnaire) about cancer being a 'socially acceptable form of suicide' didn't make sense to more than a very few in Cancer Contact. The fact remains, however, that a strong death-wish (be it for lack of love, purpose, incentive, or from a positive desire to be with someone who has already died, in the belief that there is an after-life in which we join our beloved dead) can hinder the fight against cancer. If it happens when all the odds are piling up against survival anyway, then what else can it be called but a form of suicide, which society will accept where it might condemn a deliberate overdose? But again the desire to stop living will not be enough to kill you unless the defence mechanisms have already broken down. It is said that people can worry themselves into getting cancer. In extreme cases such people sometimes take their own lives but are often found to have had no cancer at all. They were literally worried to death — but still cancer-free.

Without some obstacles human beings rarely operate effectively, and without some tension life may be no more enjoyable than an out-of-tune violin. None of us were experts, however, at keeping in tune, and Lee, who had studied relaxation with the Australian Dr Ainslie Meares (the world authority on hypnosis and relaxation) [38], taught members of the group his method and gave them foot massage. Several claimed that they had, as a result, learned to cope much more easily with everyday stress. Others found T'ai Chi or Yoga suited them better. Most of the alternative therapies described in this book were tried and proved helpful, and the spirit of the group was noticeably high. To one banished husband who had to vacate his sitting-room, the meetings sounded more like a drinks party than cancer patients discussing their problems.

Cancer was a nuisance, it could be an overwhelming nightmare, but it could not be submitted to. It had to be fought, and when we could fight no more for ourselves, we had friends who would fight for us. We were all a bit neurotic about symptoms from time to time. Was a winter 'frog in the throat' leading to throat cancer? Was a pain in the ribs a sign that cancer was now in our bones? Even an ache in the big toe had lost its innocence. There was so much to find out. O. Carl Simonton [56] said we all needed goals, and the group had provided many we had not even thought about a year before. We did not want to give up trying to live in order to make dying easier. While life lasted it must be as full and interesting and enjoyable as possible, and it was up to us to make this come about.

Cancer — What is it?

Cancer is a collection of related diseases characterised by uncontrolled growth of the body cells which are constantly mutating (changing). Every now and then they throw off a neoplasmic (cancer) cell which (if the body's defences are in good condition) will be immediately recognised as 'not-self', jumped on and destroyed. If the defences (the immune system) are not effective, then the cancer cells will multiply. Healthy cells proliferate in order to heal wounds, and they are contained and prevented from reproducing once their job is done by the collagen (gelatinous base of connective tissue) in which they are embedded. If the collagen is, however, of poor quality it will not be able to hold the cells in check; they will multiply and grow into a tumour. The quality of collagen is said to be improved by Vitamin C (see later).

There are three basic types of cancer:

1) *Carcinomas* — which are most common in adults and where the epithelial cells (cover tissues that line body cavities and glandular organs like the breast) are involved but also the mouth, lungs, prostate and gastro-intestinal tract.

2) *Sarcomas* — which are less common but highly malignant, forming in the connective tissues, muscles, bone and cartilage.

(Carcinomas and sarcomas are known as 'solid tumours'.)

3) *Leukemia* — most often found in children and caused by the over-production (and then under-production) of white blood cells. The *lymphomas* — which are found in lymphoid tissue from over-production of lymphoid cells and found in the bone marrow (from which all blood cells are thought to arise): and *multiple myelomas* — the rarest form of cancer of the bone marrow and caused by the overproduction of plasma (liquid in which the blood corpuscles float) cells.

Questionnaire

Members of Cancer Contact were asked to use the following questions as a guide in writing their case histories, the questions to be ignored or developed as they felt inclined:

Do either (or both) of your parents come from a family that gets cancer? If so, which?

When was your primary cancer first diagnosed, and where was it?

Looking back, when do *you* think it first appeared, and what were the symptoms?

If we accept that cancer doesn't suddenly appear, what would you consider the triggers? (i.e. bereavement, job dissatisfaction, domestic upheavals, difficulties with relationships, etc., also nutritional deprivation, smoking, working with chemicals, asbestos, etc.)?

Who told you that you had cancer, and how was it done (tactfully/gently/brutally, etc.)?

How many stars would you give your GP, surgeon, radiotherapist, etc. for humanity and ability to understand and succour cancer patients? (★★★★★ = first class: no stars = abysmal).

When you heard that you had cancer, were you horrified/terrified/shocked/unsurprised/despairing?

How did your family (friends, neighbours) react? Were they practical/helpful/did they try to pretend that nothing had happened/were they scared and perhaps because of this unkind, etc.?

What cancer myths (if any) did you come across (did anyone think you were infectious/bound to die just because you had 'cancer', etc.)?

What treatment were you offered and did you have?

Did you believe yourself to be 'cured' after treatment?

What advice (if any) were you given so as to remain clear of cancer in the future (i.e. re diet, smoking, work, rest, activities, etc.)?

Did you want to forget you had had cancer/take the primary as a warning of, say, 'organ inferiority' (as Adler put it)? and what steps did you take to discover how to avoid a similar cell breakdown in the future (including alternative/ complementary therapies, diet, relaxation etc.)?

What is your opinion in general, from your experience since being ill, of the treatment of cancer patients? What do you think is needed?

Why do you think you got cancer in the first place? (No answers too absurd!)

After your primaries, how often were you checked and by whom?

List briefly your illnesses before you had cancer, including operations and treatments. Do you feel that any of them were relevant to the cancer that arrived later?

Have you always been especially scared of cancer, or not?

Have you suffered a bereavement by cancer of a close relative/friend?

What do you think of the theory that there is a 'cancer personality'? (The person who gets angry inside but cannot express it, or perhaps is forbidden to do so by circumstances.) Do you feel you have much in common with other cancer sufferers which you don't have, say, with people who have other an illness or are just healthy?

How much importance do you give 'mind over matter'? Do you feel that you are in any way guilty because of cancer? (i.e. you didn't have enough faith, religion, patience, or neglected yourself while caring for others ...)

Is there anyone with whom you feel completely at

ease when discussing cancer, unorthodox methods, death, etc.?

Have you felt that even given the chance you didn't particularly want to survive, and how long did these feelings last? Cancer has been called 'a socially acceptable form of suicide'; this it obviously isn't for many, but considered coldly, do you think there is any truth in the idea?

What was your worst cancer experience, and does it help to talk/write about it? Can it be used to help others?

How difficult have you found these questions?

Secondary cancers:

How long after the primaries did they appear?

What symptoms, if any, did you suspect/report/have treated, which might have been recognised as secondary cancer?

If you were told you were cured of cancer at the primary stage, did this, do you think, make it difficult for your GP to admit to you (or himself) that your symptoms were serious?

How were the secondaries discovered? (By your GP/in hospital, and if so, how ... by X-ray/biopsy/etc.?)

Who told you that you had secondary cancer and how was it done (tactfully/brutally/casually etc.)? Were you given time to discuss the situation?

Were you alone? If not, how was your husband/wife/ friend informed?

Were you given any prognosis? Did you ask for one? If so, how and what were you told?

If the news was bad, were you given comfort/encouragement to survive/practical advice re diet/etc. etc.?

What treatment (if any) were you offered? What did you agree to have?

What, if anything, did you refuse to do or have?

Did you consider or turn to alternative therapies, homoeopathy, etc? If so, how did your GP/surgeon/consultant react? Did they all co-operate/insist that only they had the answer/denigrate methods other than their own/get in touch with your 'second opinion'? And how content/worried/unhappy were you about the progress of your battle against cancer?

What was your greatest problem: pain/anxiety/depression/terror for your nearest and dearest? Could you communicate about any of these and with whom? If you took remedies to ease all or some of these problems, what were they?

How long is it now since your secondaries were diagnosed, and how does it go?

II. Ten Patients' Stories

The following autobiographical stories from cancer patients (all members of Cancer Contact) are in order of their ages, which range from 32 to 67. Names have been changed so that all contributors could express themselves freely.

★

Kathleen was born in 1950. She was too poorly to write her own account but tape recorded the following story of her cancer and the life that led up to it.

My parents both came from Eire but I was born in Sheffield. I was the second child and have a sister two and a half years older than me, but my mother also had a lot of miscarriages. When my brother was born my mother and father separated. I have only one recollection of him while we were all together. He was a tractor driver and was killed when his tractor drove over a pipe which somehow hit him and split his head open. After that we three children lived with my mother in bed-sitters on National Assistance. I had started going to a local country school.

When I was seven my uncle tried to rape both my sister and myself. She told my mother and we never saw him again. I think we had been quite fond of him. Then my mother met a man twelve years younger than she was and they married. This was OK for a while, but they found three kids difficult and he decided he wanted my sister and me to go and live in Ireland, while just my brother stayed at home. We were to go to my auntie, but when my mother took us over to Ireland, she couldn't bring herself to leave us there and so back we came again.

There were awful fights between my mother and stepfather: once she sliced him with a knife and he threw a brick into her face. I took my blouse off to try to stop the bleeding. He wasn't a basically bad man, but there were endless rows. Once he sold most of our furniture.

In 1958 we all moved into a proper house in Corby. Mother was always telling my sister not to argue and praising me because I was so quiet. My brother and I had withdrawn into a dream world of our own. Of course my sister was jealous, always hearing about how good I was. One day I found my mother lying in the street with her head split open and her ribs broken. My stepfather was unconscious lying in a pool of blood in the hallway where she had half-killed him. It was about then, I think, that she had found a letter from some other woman who had had his baby.

After this we were a fatherless family with all the stigma that is attached. I wasn't particularly bright at school, but I wasn't dim. I only half-listened from my dream world, and had occasional bursts of temper.

I wanted to do hairdressing when I left school at 15. I couldn't though, because when my sister had wanted to go to secretarial college my mother had told her she had to go out to work, so of course she objected to the idea of my getting an apprenticeship. So I went to work for a chemist who was an officious bitch of a woman, though she may have had her reasons. I had no qualifications, of course. My stepfather returned for a while, but things still went badly between him and my mother. Then I went to work in a shoe factory, and when I was 16 my sister and I left home. I always had friends; one boyfriend and I were close for three years or so. There were four of us sharing a bed-sitter, then my sister left. Someone took my alarm clock, so I was often late for work. I didn't have enough money to buy another one.

I had one steady boyfriend who wanted to marry me, but when I became pregnant I went back home. I lost the baby just before my 17th birthday. I was four months pregnant. My mother was out at bingo. I was losing blood for about an hour. I lost six pints. When my mother came home she nearly hit the roof. All she could say was 'What will the neighbours say?' — the same neighbours who had seen *her* lying in the road! It was an hour or so before she got an ambulance for me.

When I was 18 I got engaged and moved with my boyfriend down to Sussex, but after a while I told him I didn't want to live with him any more.

My mother was a very tough lady. She died of heart trouble in 1976, after several strokes. I found that the death of my cat two years before had been a much more painful experience for me than her death. I was distraught about my cat and cried for days. It nearly broke my heart.

I met Sue in 1971 and we were to share a home for 11 years, but although I couldn't live without her, I also couldn't live with her. It was in 1979 that I went to my GP about a very heavy menstrual discharge with periods every two weeks. He took swift action. At 2.30 one afternoon in April I was given a smear test and by 3.00 I was in hospital where they gave me a D & C. I give my doctor ★★★★. When I was told that I had cancer of the cervix I was quite upset. Not horrified, but quite upset. My friends were very helpful and good. No one said that I would never get cancer again, but I understood that it was all cleared up. No one gave me any advice as to how to look after myself.

I was 31 in February 1982 when I found a gland on my neck and was given a general anaesthetic for a biopsy. Although I was told that the gland was malignant, it wasn't until December that I really discovered that I had secondary cancer. I had to have radiotherapy which caused me a lot of pain. I was driving myself to and from hospital while I was sitting my examination for the National Certificate of Horticulture (Nursery Practice). I was very pleased when I passed, but none of my teachers seemed to realise how much it had cost me, and how much effort I had had to make to keep my studies and the treatment going at the same time. They didn't even seem very pleased with my result.

My consultant wanted me to have chemotherapy. When I refused she washed her hands of me and wouldn't make any more suggestions or co-operate. Meanwhile I had seen a leaflet in the local church about the Mid-Sussex Homoeopathic Group, and I fixed up an appointment with a homoeopathic doctor who put me onto Iscador injections and gave me other remedies which were effective in dealing with my symptoms. I felt much better while I was having the Iscador and quite down on the days when I didn't.

During 1982 things became quite impossible with Sue. I became completely depressed and gave up having my injections and never remembered to take my vitamins or anything. I was going to bed without washing myself and putting on the same clothes day after day. I was really desperate. My memory of this time is confused, but I know that one day I cut up all Sue's clothes. She and my GP took me to the local mental hospital, and in the car park I got my hands round her throat. I think I wanted to kill her. A wonderful psychiatric nurse helped me and took me in. But all the hospital could do was to prescribe drugs, and I didn't want them. I stayed there two weeks.

Sue and I sold our house, and she left the district. I had nowhere to live, and tried everywhere to get a job on a farm, or in a nursery. I rented a caravan for a while and then divided my time between my sister and a friend who is said to be a manic-depressive. She says she is much happier since she was 'saved for Jesus' by the Pentecostalists. She wanted me to join them, and for a while I thought it might be the answer. But I think I was using religion only as an escape. I needed to think a lot more about it.

After my last visit to Sue I knew our relationship was all over. She had gone to pieces. I felt really free again. I washed my hair and did my face and went to my new GP; I had left the other one as he wasn't co-operative about alternatives to orthodox treatment and didn't have time to spend on my problems. I felt really good and free at last. Then he told me that the result of the latest X-rays showed that the cancer was now in my spine. I cried such a lot all the mascara ran down my face. I don't know why my spine wasn't investigated before. They also said I have a shadow round my pelvis, but they didn't tell me what it is. I started having a great deal of pain and was quite fuzzy with all the painkillers I was taking. My friend says I am too meek and, when I couldn't get a doctor to come to me in the night, she said I should get angry, so I did. 'Thank you for nothing,' I said, and rang off. He rang me back, and then came and gave me an injection and stayed to talk. He was really good. Every day I felt totally exhausted.

This lasted quite a while, then — thanks to Lee, the State Registered Nurse who is the mainstay of the cancer group — I started having Iscador injections again. She came to give them to me whenever I needed them, and also drove me about and had me to stay for the day at her home every week. She was wonderful. I also found the meetings of Cancer Contact a tremendous help: I feel so relieved. It's lovely to see all the girls.

Lee put me in touch with a healer, and it's perhaps his help (or the Jason Winters' tea, or the strong doses of Vitamin C or the injections) that are beginning to help a little and remove some of the swelling from my leg and feet. Now I am going into a local hospice for a couple of weeks to get a rest. I really do need a rest. There is so much tension, and I don't seem to be able to take it any more ... and I still grieve for Sue.

I think that when I first got cancer I felt it was terminal and I was fatalistic about it. That's where I started to go wrong, because I didn't fight. Although I have been a vegetarian for a long time, until recently no one gave me any other advice about how to keep fit. I realise now that I didn't change my way of life enough to stay healthy.

The mental hospital had been unable to do anything for Kathleen's depression and when she came out she had no home of her own to go to. She accepted Lee's invitation to go and live with her but with some misgivings: there had been so many rejections. How long could she put up with her? She decided it was worth the risk and moved in. For Kathleen's last months Lee looked after her day and night with loving care and professional nursing skill, giving up her own bedroom and sharing everything with Kathleen. Members of Cancer Contact visited them both, not out of duty but because by now there was genuine friendship and concern. Kathleen's fight for life continued to be spasmodic: sometimes she lost heart, refused her injections and said she wished it were all over, but at other times she continued to take an interest in everyone, learning how to do patchwork and talking of taking music lessons. Lee bought her a descant recorder and read her the Bible in the evenings. Cancer Contact gave a tea-party when Kathleen was able to go out into the garden and see the spring bulbs flowering. We planned further visits when the weather was warmer.

Kathleen became steadily more disabled and when Lee could no longer cope alone, Kathleen went back to the Hospice. Here her brother, sister and friends visited her. Kathleen's days were spent drifting between confusion, lucidity and unconsciousness, and it was difficult to tell if her hallucinations were part of the disease or the effect of drugs which were relieving most of her pain. She died at the age of 32, in June 1983. Cancer Contact had lost a friend and their first member. Their arrangements of garden and wild flowers accompanied the coffin.

Kathleen's dying had been nearly as traumatic as her life and there were many questions now for the group to discuss, such as the rights of a very confused patient, the wishes of medically uninformed relatives and friends, and the judgment of the GP and nursing staff. It is a question of trust: do we trust our next of kin to choose wisely? Do we want our doctors to decide what is best for us even if in opposition to our family? These are decisions which perhaps we should face before the traumas can arise. It was a subject for Cancer Contact to wrestle with.

★

Mary was born in 1946. Her mother's family have all died of cancer. She was 35 when she first noticed a breast lump.

I feel it had probably been there some time. By the time the primary cancer was discovered, it had already established secondaries in the lymph nodes. This was a severe blow to my pride, as I have always been what my family call 'a bit cranky' about my health. I don't smoke, or drink. I eat a high-fibre, almost vegetarian diet, walk miles because I have no car, and take a large daily dose of vitamin pills and ginseng.

My husband had to break the news to me about the results of the biopsy, although he had been promised that the surgeon would tell me himself, before my husband came to see me. The first I knew of the bad news was my husband's extreme state of distress when he arrived at my bedside. We were joined fairly soon by the surgeon, who was brief and to-the-point, and told me that I had an early carcinoma of the breast. He advised an immediate mastectomy.

My GP gets no stars at all! He had been unconcerned two years before when I consulted him about the very swollen gland in my armpit, was fairly casual about the lump in my breast, and refused to visit me at home when I came out of hospital, full of worries and anxieties which I badly needed to discuss. My surgeon gets ★★ because he was, in the end, very thorough in his discussions with us about my treatment and completely honest about my prognosis. Although he was encouraging about my post-operative progress, in the days immediately following my operation he was always too busy and rushed to answer my questions, making me feel slightly foolish and neurotic. But on the whole I found him kind. The doctor in charge of the radiotherapy gets ★★★★★. I went to him determined not to have his beastly treatment, and he must have spent an hour telling me in great detail exactly why I should have it, what might happen if I didn't, what my chances were, and answering all my doubts and queries with infinite sympathy and patience. In all my subsequent dealings with him he was equally gentle, humane and reasonable, and was most co-operative about letting me use homoeopathic creams and remedies.

My family was absolutely wonderful. My husband has been my greatest support, despite his own moments of pessimism and despair. Parents and sister were wonderfully compassionate, completely practical and immensely helpful. Friends rallied round and were unbelievably helpful and kind, taking over the children, helping my parents, making meals, etc. and later on driving me to Brighton for radiotherapy. A few friends were embarrassingly over-emotional, and *everyone* rushed off in a panic for tests, screenings and examinations! Two or three friends behaved as if I must be on my way out, and one in particular makes it quite clear that she thinks I am dying. She herself has a pathological dread of cancer. Only my next-door neighbour behaved as if very little had happened.

I was offered: mastectomy, radiotherapy to the affected area, radiation menopause (to remove oestrogen), Tamoxifen, and steroids, with plastic surgery to follow later on. I refused only the steroids, and in addition I consulted a homoeopathic doctor who prescribed Iscador injections. I have had to discontinue these because of the severe local reaction and pain they caused, but I believe they helped me through my radiotherapy.

I didn't imagine I was 'cured' after these treatments, but believed that I was temporarily out of danger. I felt it was up to me to try to work out why this had happened to me, and felt that, hopefully, this would prevent a recurrence.

No one gave me any advice whatsoever with regard to diet or lifestyle at this time. It took me some while to get a doctor to admit to me that the investigation of my lymph gland (at the same time as the removal of the primary) had revealed secondary growths. My surgeon merely told me, after he received my histology, that the lymph glands were affected, 'But that's all gone, so it doesn't matter'. Later, when I understood more about the subject, I asked the consultant radiotherapist how exactly the lymph gland had been affected. He told me that two of the nodes had growths around them, and when I asked if these would be secondaries, he very gently and almost reluctantly confirmed this. I was given the prognosis ten days after the operation and biopsy. My surgeon told me that he would like to say I was cured but that would be neither fair nor true. He said I had a 50 per cent chance of survival for the next five years. It was conceivable, however, that the cancer had already spread to my shoulder, and a recurrence was most likely in the first two years. He spoke to my husband first, to find out whether I should be told, then told me alone, and then repeated the whole thing with my husband present. With proper treatment and luck, he said, I might be one of the fortunate 50 per cent. He would do everything possible for me, in view of my youth, and he was optimistic about my chances because I had been such an excellent patient so far.

When I told my GP that I was considering homoeopathic treatment instead of radiotherapy, he listened quite patiently to my reasons and agreed to prescribe it for me, although he said that, as an orthodox doctor, he could not encourage me in this. He suggested that before I came to any firm decision I should consult my radiotherapist, who agreed that no one had the answer or the cure, that the decision had to be mine alone, and that he didn't envy it. He also said that if there *were* a cancer treatment that made you feel well, had no side effects and actually worked, then I could be sure he would use it himself! He did not denigrate homoeopathy, merely regretted its lack of proper clinical trials.

In the end I decided to have both orthodox and homoeopathic treatment, as my family were so anxious for me to have the former, and then met with a considerable lack of encouragement from my GP although one of his junior partners was kind and co-operative. My GP refused to make it easy for me to have the injections, was unsympathetic about the pain I had with them ('Well, nobody's asking you to have them') and implied that it was all a waste of time anyway. As a result of this experience I changed GPs, and my new doctor is quite happy to prescribe Iscador for me, should I want it, and feels that a patient should have the final say in what treatment is administered. He has spent patient hours discussing my worries, queries, theories etc., and has lent me self-help books such as *Getting Well Again*. I now feel that some progress is being made in my own battle.

My greatest problem, apart from pain and discomfort which were dominant for a few weeks, was facing the fact that I had a life-threatening disease and that I might not see my children grow up. Fortunately I can talk about this to my husband, and we have had matter-of-fact discussions about the possibility of my death and how he would face it. My parents are unwilling to discuss this and take the attitude that 'It's not going to happen'. I have never taken any drugs for depression about the future (or to kill pain) and find that my now strong belief in my own powers of recovery and health are the best antidote to fear of an early death.

Looking back, I consider that the 'triggers' started when I was 28 in 1974, with the break-up of my first marriage and helped along by my high-pressure job (journalism, with all its deadlines and competitiveness) and my own inability to be on time for anything, which gave me a constantly churning stomach! In 1976 I re-married and had two children in quick succession. Between them they gave me not *one* unbroken night for five years. They were difficult babies and toddlers, and I am not a naturally maternal person. Add to that a husband who in those days was moody and critical, and a very busy lifestyle — always trying to do too much in too little time! — and you have a perfect recipe for stress and the resulting suppression of the immune system leading to cancer. I am certain that my body's defences were not working properly, because in the two years preceding the diagnosis I was constantly unwell. Despite the health care I have already mentioned, I had one infection or virus following another, and I was never free of unusually bad colds, coughs, throat infections, mouth ulcers, thrush and other small miseries. Generally speaking I have had none of these since May 1982.

I don't find it possible to forget that I have had cancer, but I do get bored by constantly thinking about it, discussing it and adapting my life to it. I have tried to read as much as possible on the subject to find out where I may have gone wrong, and am now practising the methods which seem to make sense. I am even more purist about my diet and vitamins, have tried to cut out the stressful elements of my life, slow down a bit, care more about my own needs and feelings, and practise relaxation.

Cancer Contact has been helping not only in suggesting alternative therapies and remedies, but also in providing moral support and contact with other determined cancer patients. Lee has not only taught us the importance of complete relaxation, but has also showed us how to practise it, with a foot massage technique which affects the well-being of the whole body.

I think there may be something in the argument that there is a specific cancer personality. I am convinced that my own trigger was stress. I have always had difficulty in expressing anger or aggression, and I constantly suppress these feelings. But other people who have no such repressions also get cancer, presumably for other reasons, depending on the type of cancer and the prevailing circumstances. I don't feel that I have anything more in common with cancer patients than with other people, apart from having cancer.

I believe very strongly in the ability of the mind to influence one's physical state. I don't feel any guilt over what has happened so far, as I had no idea the harm stress can cause. I don't regret any of my past life, but I've no doubt that I will feel very guilty if I do get a recurrence, as I now believe that I have far more control over my health than I ever realised.

I have never at any point felt that I did not want to go on living, although this may be because of my age and the fact that I have two small children. My survival instinct has always been very strong and has carried me through many a crisis in my life. I therefore find it very hard to accept the idea of cancer as a form of suicide. I do believe, however, that the will to live is vital in conquering any disease and I know that many people, when they discover they have cancer, just sit back and wait for death to come.

The worst aspect of cancer to me has undoubtedly been the loss of the breast; both the pain and discomfort (which are still with me), and the feeling of being mutilated and 'damaged'. Despite my husband's wonderful attitude towards it, I find it very hard to reconcile myself to the loss. This plus my unnaturally early radiation menopause, and the awful finality of not being able to have any more children, have combined to make me feel that cancer has not only robbed me of my health, but has also spoiled my womanhood. This is something that, oddly enough, most of my friends find hard to understand — so talking about it doesn't help much. They only say 'But you don't *look* any different', and even my husband feels that losing a breast and ovaries is terribly unimportant compared to being alive.

I think cancer patients, generally speaking, are not given sufficient information and advice on their condition. They need time to talk, which the average GP cannot give. Too many people seem to be given treatment or drugs without any explanation of what they are supposed to do. I often wonder how I would have fared, had I not pestered, asked questions, sought alternatives, and finally changed my GP. Nobody seems at all interested in one's background, lifestyle, diet habits, etc., which makes me wonder what cancer research is all about. A standard questionnaire to cancer patients ought to be routine, possibly followed up by specific advice on how to prevent a recurrence. What is really needed are nation-wide cancer clinics, giving unbiased facts about all the different methods of cancer treatment; their pros and cons, their success rates, etc.

At the beginning of 1983, eight months after the mastectomy, I went into hospital for what is called 'breast reconstruction'. This is a major operation, available on the NHS, in which the large muscle from the back, and the skin above it, are moved round to the front to create a breast mound. On opening up the back, they found that radiotherapy had considerably atrophied the muscle, so it was necessary to put in a small saline implant beneath the transplanted muscle, to bulk it out.

The operation, four hours of it, involved a ten-day

stay in hospital and a fair amount of pain and discomfort for the first few days, because I had surgery front and back. But as with childbirth, I felt I was going to gain something at the end of it all, which helped me to put up with all the drips, drains, and minor miseries. On the fifth day, when the bandages were changed and I gazed at my miraculously soft and pillowy chest, I realised that it had been worth every twinge. The result, apart from two elliptical scars, is almost identical to what I lost, and makes me feel a whole person again. The feeling of having been mutilated has completely gone, and I no longer think 'I've had cancer' every time I get undressed.

Throughout the post-operative weeks I was sustained, as before, by the loving support of all the family, and by my faith in my own ability to survive, as well as a sort of martyred pride in coping heroically! I found that I was spurred on to greater efforts of activity by wanting badly to be able to do things, such as my drawing and painting, gardening, bread-making — even my own housework! Now one year after the cancer diagnosis, I can truly say that I feel not only quite back to normal, but also that the quality of my life has improved.

★

Sheila was born in 1943, when her mother was 42. Neither of her parents, and none of her relations, had had cancer. The first symptom she noticed was a slight discolouration on the side of her breast in 1977.

My GP thought it was a blood vessel. A year later I saw his senior partner for advice about the pill, and he noticed nothing wrong until I pointed it out. He then sent me to the surgeon on a Friday. The surgeon arranged for an immediate mammograph, and the next day phoned me to say that although it appeared to be

OK, he thought there was a slight puckering of the breast. He asked me to attend the Outpatients at the local hospital on the Monday for a biopsy. I worried about this for the whole weekend as I did not understand how you could have a biopsy in Outpatients! It turned out that they had wanted me to go into hospital the next day, but they only had a room off the men's ward, which I did not fancy, and as the children were just about to go back to school, I left it another week. I then went into hospital. I went privately, as my husband belonged to BUPA through his office. I also thought it would hurry things along, and this was important as we were probably going to have to move house very soon.

My surgeon told me that he did not think there was any malignancy, but that if he found there was, he would have to remove my breast. The night before the operation I was asked to sign a form in which I agreed to a mastectomy if it proved necessary. I waited before signing it until my husband came in. It did not hit him until then, which somehow upset me more than anything. He asked if a second opinion could not be had before removing the breast, but this was refused.

The next morning I came out of the anaesthetic to see the surgeon's assistant at my bedside. I asked him if it had been removed, and he said 'yes'. I do not remember anything else being said to me. I was, it seemed, quite heavily sedated. I sat up in bed, feeling sick and hardly able to open my eyes. I accepted the diagnosis philosophically; I had had my upset the night before.

I do not think any of my family really wanted to speak with me about cancer. Although they all lived some distance away, some of them did manage to come and see me. My father had died in 1975 after several strokes; he had been terribly Victorian and I think I probably married to get away from him. My mother was now 78. I think my sister was worried that she might also get cancer after my experience, for she made several trips to see her doctor. She is fourteen years older than I am, and my brother twelve years older. I was the misfit! I don't think anybody wanted to speak about my experience, and I believe that my mother-in-law (who was looking after the girls, then aged eight and six) was sure I would die just because I had cancer.

Three weeks after the radical mastectomy and removal of the lymph gland, I was sterilised. It was five months before I was given radiotherapy 'as a precaution'. Then I had 18 months of chemotherapy, first by injection and then orally, from 1979 to 1980. In June 1980 I was given a scan and told I should have one every two years. I was to have regular checks, but you were usually believed to be OK after five years. I think I was told to cut down on smoking (although I did not smoke a lot) and that swimming was good for me, but I didn't pay a lot of attention because I just wanted to forget I had had cancer.

A few weeks before Xmas 1980 I fell downstairs, and I thought this was the cause of an ache in my groin at this time. My GP said it might be a hernia, although this was unusual in women. He gave me some exercises to do. In January 1981 I was due to see the surgeon. A nurse at the hospital noticed that I was limping and told me to report it, and when I did I was sent immediately for X-rays. I then had four different courses of radiotherapy, starting with the groin. I was so raw after two weeks that I was sent to the skin reaction clinic. I also had radiotherapy to the pelvis and back and was given drugs for the sickness. My ovaries were burned out and I hoped that this would stop the growth, but it didn't. The radiotherapist wanted me to have more chemotherapy, but the surgeon thought I was too young at 38. He wanted to remove my pituitary gland. So I saw the ENT specialist, who explained how it would be taken out from the front of the brain through the side of the nose. As I was leaving, he told me that I had no choice. The operation had to be done to stop the pain and prevent the cancer from growing.

After being tested for different allergies, I had the gland removed on June 30th, 1981, and awoke with a large patch over my right eye and my nose literally stuffed with wadding. I had to wear nose bolsters because it was running all the time. Three days later I went down with pneumonia. The ENT surgeon was away at a conference, and it wasn't until a few days later that I realised that none of his assistants had ever seen the operation before. The nursing sister put a fan to cool me, and ice on my neck. When one of the assistants tried to insert a drip into my arm he caused me so much pain that I complained. He then slung it down and walked out on me! Someone else tried a different drip.

I was in a room to myself for two weeks and felt very lonely. There were only rooftops and chimneys to look at out of the window. I was glad when they agreed to transfer me nearer home. It was lovely to see the green grass again. Again the staff had not come across a case like mine before, but one of the nurses tried to read up about it and understand to the best of her ability. I had to make a fuss when they produced terribly old-fashioned nasal sprays. My temperature was still going up a lot, but the surgeons seemed pleased with me. Then they put me on valium. I felt terrible from then on, not knowing quite what I was doing and feeling unsafe on my feet, so I asked for it to be stopped. I was in hospital for another two weeks.

My first evening back home, and every evening from then on my husband was out. Of course, he had to shop and cook. I couldn't do anything much. By the end of a week, the district nurse and I both thought I would have to go back into hospital because I was feeling so rotten. Everything had gone wrong with my digestion. I was taking Cortisone Acetate. Without it I knew I would go into a coma. I was also taking sleeping pills, and pills for the pain, and Nolvadex (Tamoxifen) and quite a few others. One of the side effects was thrush on my tongue and gums. During that summer (1981) my surgeon said that I should have some X-rays taken to see if the removal of my pituitary gland had worked as he hoped. My GP couldn't remember which were the relevant parts for X-raying so he asked for me to be X-rayed from my toes to my head. I found this very strange. I don't believe in having unnecessary radiation.

I can't remember who told me that I had secondary cancer. I think I had guessed it because of the rush they were in to have me X-rayed. I don't think I was given any prognosis. They seemed to think that radiotherapy would do the trick, but in fact it made me feel very low. The radiotherapist wanted me to have chemotherapy, but I would have lost my hair. I was so upset that they sent me to see a social worker, who began to give me details of how to get a wig.

In July 1982 my right arm and hand became terribly swollen. I had understood from a book that this might happen. I'd been careful not to have any needles in that arm, or have it used to take my blood pressure unless it was absolutely essential. My GP said that I was lucky not to have had this problem before, and that there was nothing that could help it. I asked for some physiotherapy which I had read about and, although he knew nothing about it himself, he arranged it for me. Now, five months later, the swelling is no better. The Mastectomy Association suggested a machine made by Talley Ltd, which has helped a lot of people, but the physios don't seem to be interested. I have given them details, but they say that anyway there is no money for such things! I'm sure that there would be lots of other people who could benefit from it. I'm going to ask my surgeon if he can help. The arm doesn't hurt, but it's heavy and a nuisance as I can't wear blouses, or do up my cuffs, and my hand is very clumsy. I still do not know the reason why it suddenly became so swollen.

After joining the Mid-Sussex Homoeopathic Group I went to see a homoeopathic doctor. He said he wouldn't prescribe Iscador as I was already taking quite enough drugs. He explained that the dry skin and cuts on my hands were the result of hormone imbalance, and he seemed to know all about the operation I had had. The drops he gave me don't appear to have done my arm any good, but my hands are a little better.

I have been trying to learn relaxation but I find it very difficult. I cannot do visualisation therapy for if I shut my eyes I cannot even 'see' my daughters' faces. I am now taking 2-4 grams of Vitamin C every day but if I take too much I get a lot of flatulence. The Dr Bach flower remedies really do seem to help me to cope better. A homoeopathic consultant gave me Calendula ointment for my hands, Calc. Fluor for my bones and Apis and Stannum for the lymphodaemia. I haven't talked to my GP about homoeopathy as I don't think he agrees with it. My surgeon also doesn't think much of it, although he says it couldn't do me any harm. He didn't want me to take any extra vitamins.

I have tried not to think any more about cancer. I think my unhappy marriage upset me more than my illness. Until recently I couldn't talk to my children, but now that they are 14 and 12 we do discuss cancer sometimes. I don't want them to have their father's problems with communication. The district nurse was very understanding and concerned about the pain, but I couldn't even tell her how near I felt I had been to death.

Every day I have to take cortisone morning and evening, and more frequently if I feel I am catching a cold or something. I have to take Thyroxine twice a day for my thyroid as a result of losing my pituitary gland and I still take Nolvadex. I also have to measure carefully my water intake and output so that I know whether or not to use the nasal spray. I believe that domestic upheavals and so many moves helped to trigger my cancer. We first moved house two months after we married in 1965. My daughters were born in 1968 and 1971. I couldn't breast-feed them. Although I had enough milk, it wasn't reaching the babies for some reason. In 1971 we moved to Bristol. We seemed always to be having to move because of my husband's changes of jobs. When my husband went on ahead of us to Sussex, our marriage radically took a turn for the worse as his social life became more important to him. He still very rarely returns home before midnight. Then he was made redundant and it was likely the children would have to go to a state school but we managed to avoid this.

I joined the Mid-Sussex Homoeopathic Group through meeting the person who started it, and who kindly visited me a lot in hospital. Another friend had also spoken of the group and was interested in joining. Since then Cancer Contract has been formed, and I find this most helpful. We have many things in common and are able to chat as much as we like about ourselves. This is a relief, as I am sure our healthy friends do not like to hear too much about our problems. We also hear of others trying different homoeopathic remedies, which in turn makes us feel more inclined to use them. I also learned about Vitamin C and Jason Winters' tea, and how they can help you to fight cancer. I am sure that they helped ease the little pain which I was left with after my last operation.

★

Gordon was born in 1939. He writes:

Ever since my mother died of cancer when I was 20 I have been scared of it. My father has had cancer of the throat for the last five years. My own bowel cancer was first diagnosed in April 1983. For eighteen months my

GP had been treating me for indigestion: 'advertising tummy' is what he called it. I give him minus nil stars. He was hopeless. At last I insisted on seeing a specialist in stomach and bowel diseases paying for the barium enema and the operation myself. I could have gone into hospital on the NHS but frankly don't believe NHS staff could have coped with my need of a bedpan every five minutes. I feel that if I hadn't insisted on going private I would probably be dead.

It was the specialist who, in answer to my question, told me that I had cancer. He was very much to the point — but how does one define 'brutally'? I give both my surgeon and radiotherapist ★★★★★. I was horrified and terrified by the diagnosis, although I was not surprised. I had been taking it for granted that there was a possibility that I would get cancer ever since my mother died.

My family and friends were fantastically practical and helpful, but of course they were scared. My wife has been marvellous. I was, however, given no advice whatsoever by the hospital as to how to avoid cancer in the future. I was told that the tumour had been removed but that there were some rogue cancer cells that had to be treated by chemotherapy. Now, in August 1983, I am still attending the Marsden Hospital and having their special 'freezing' treatment in order to keep my hair.

I have, since April, contacted every recognised cancer organisation there is, but all to no avail. I am absolutely disgusted and horrified by their lack of interest in prevention and the fact that with all the money they get as charities, none goes for research into alternative therapies. They are only interested in you if you are dying.

Cancer Contact (which I joined with the Mid-Sussex Homoeopathic Group) has been very helpful. I can't say yet which of all the therapies I am trying (from diet and hypnosis to acupuncture) are going to prove successful. I shall have to wait and see. Meanwhile my biggest problem is learning how to relax and I am going to get in touch with Lee to see if she can help.

I believe that there *is* a cancer personality and that cancer is caused by stress. My own stress was all part of my job in advertising. Before all this I had never had a day's illness although I did neglect my health. My inability to relax must have been a major cause of my own cancer.

For me, any questions about my attitudes to death are unnecessary. I don't want to discuss it. I do feel benefit, however, from being able to talk about cancer, especially with other people who have been through some of the same experiences. I no longer say that I am completely cured, but I know I have defeated the cancer. I have no religious beliefs but I am sure that mind does have a strong influence over matter and I am determined to be fit. I am already putting on some weight.

Without being disrespectful I think there should have been at least another 10-20 questions in the questionnaire. I am quite sure that there should be more after-care for cancer patients: at the moment hospitals provide none at all. I continue to pay privately for my treatments and it is all very expensive. However I have managed to get my vitamins and food supplements (including Amygdalin) on the NHS and hope that other members of Cancer Contact will be able to do the same.

★

Daphne was born in 1934. None of her own family had had cancer. Her mother-in-law, however, died of it (in the oesophagus) in 1972. She had complained for many years about not being able to eat, swallow and digest food properly, but had been treated only for 'nerves'. It was only just before her death that her illness has correctly diagnosed.

My own primary cancer was first diagnosed in March 1978, and I had a segmental mastectomy of the left breast. I was horrified, terrified, shocked and despairing. I told my husband and our vicar that as I looked outside and saw all the spring flowers coming through, I felt that next spring I would be pushing them up! I was in a state of severe shock for weeks after and cried constantly. My (young) GP was too complacent for words. He never came to see me when I returned home to convalesce — and he even bungled a prescription for cotton wool! When my husband and I tackled him, he assured us that he had never 'let anyone slip through the net before' and that, all being well, he would give me at least another ten years! I decided to change my GP immediately and to go to another practice in the area. This proved difficult and I had to write a letter explaining why I wanted to change. In this, I was completely frank about my reasons — and was informed that I had been accepted.

My family and friends and neighbours (especially those from our church) were all marvellous and supportive. Everyone was practical and helpful, listening when I did the talking and not trying to pretend that nothing had happened to me. I had always believed that cancer was a death sentence. My mother, bless her, said once that perhaps I had 'got it' from my mother-in-law as 'no one in our family had ever had it'!

Looking back, I think the first symptom appeared in August 1977, as a pea-like lump pressing on my rib-cage. I consulted my GP about it but he didn't think it was anything serious and said it was probably just a cyst that would go of its own accord. There was no question of my seeing anyone else about it, as far as he was concerned, although I was at the surgery almost every day at that time, because our six-year-old son had a fairly serious disorder of the colon and was needing constant medical attention. A couple of months later I mentioned that I still had the lump, but again my GP expressed no concern. Eventually, my mother came to stay and came with me to the doctor about our son, whose condition was now very serious. Our male GP was away, and instead we saw his (female) locum. On seeing the ghastly bagful of laundry I had taken in support of my plea that my son be referred, she wrote immediately to a paediatrician. When my husband and I took the boy to see him, he expressed his horror of the enemas and manipulation our GP had been giving. These treatments 'went out with the ark', he said, and completely changed the handling of the case.

In March 1978, I returned to our GP and again asked about the lump in my breast, which was growing more palpable. We were shortly going to move house and I wanted my mounting anxiety dispelled before becoming immersed in the move. Now he had to agree to writing a letter of referral to a consultant. Within 48 hours, I had an appointment with him at the hospital, and was advised to have surgery straight away. I told the surgeon that I didn't think I could come in for a week or so, as our son was in hospital and I had rather a lot on, with my duties as a magistrate on the local Bench. He told me that all those things could go on without me, but we could wait just over the weekend.

On the Monday morning we arrived at an unusually quiet hospital, the staff having been very badly hit by a particularly severe strain of flu. A 'red warning' was in force; no patients were being admitted. My admission, however, seemed to be an exception, for the whole theatre staff were ready for me. I felt very worried at all the fuss, and began thinking that I would feel very stupid if the lump proved to be nothing at all. I learned later that immediately this was removed, its colour indicated that it was a malignant carcinoma. It was rushed to Pathology at another hospital, with a police escort, while I remained in the theatre, and the result was telephoned back. By this time, however, I had been under the anaesthetic for some time and it was decided to stitch me up and take counsel all round.

When the surgeon came into my room later that day, I was dozing. I heard him saying that he would come back when I was awake, as I 'wouldn't understand'. That was quite enough to rouse me! I told him I was wide awake. The next day, there was a conference round my bed: the surgeon and his colleagues, my husband and me. I was told that they wanted to operate again, the following morning, for further 'excavation'; then I was to have radiotherapy. We agreed to all these suggestions. My surgeon gets ★★★★★ while my former GP no stars at all! My consultant radiotherapist only ★★★★, because he did not tell me about the overall and lasting effects of radiation.

In December 1980, just as we were again about to move house from Surrey to Sussex, I noticed a slight discharge from my right nipple. I wasn't unduly concerned, as all the tests, throughout March and April (blood,mammography,etc.) proved negative, and the surgeon said that it was a blocked milk duct. He said that, nevertheless, he wasn't going to take any chances with me and wanted to operate immediately.

This time, it was the May Bank Holiday and the histology laboratory was closed, so I was discharged and sent home. I returned to hospital ten days later for the removal of the sutures when, as before, my surgeon told me the news in the presence of the consultant radiotherapist. It was a second cancer — not a 'secondary' but another primary. I was given time, there and then, to discuss everything. Once again, I readily agreed to radiotherapy. I did not honestly think that there were any alternatives, but even if I had known of any I would probably still have made the same decisions, as I felt radiotherapy to be positive follow-through treatment.

In August 1981, I had a suspicious lump removed from my left leg. Happily, this was found not to be malignant. I imagined, erroneously, that the more time that passed, the better my chances. Eventually I believed myself to be 'cured'. Indeed, at one of my check-ups, my surgeon said that he did not think I would have any further cancer.

Of course, I haven't been able to forget that I have had it, but no one — at GP level — gave me either advice on how to stay well, encouragement to survive or practical advice about diet, etc.

My greatest problem was anxiety, depression and terror for my nearest and dearest. I was able to talk about this at *any* time with my husband. The only drugs I took were to help me sleep; after both operations, I was unable to sleep properly at night for a year.

Now, at the beginning of 1983, I have an external breast 'pimple'. I have been told by my surgeon to go straight back to his Cancer Clinic at the hospital if it doesn't go. It was bleeding in December 1982. As it has subsided, I shall wait now until March. I am examined every three months by my surgeon and consultant radiotherapist at a Joint Cancer Clinic at the hospital where I had my surgery, but if I find anything suspicious, I have immediate access to my surgeon and consultant radiotherapist, bypassing my GP. I am worried, however, that I may not be so lucky as to get 'warnings', if there is a next time. But, as my surgeon has said, I have really been very lucky. Unfortunately, I am terribly vulnerable to virus infections and succumb to one kind or another every few weeks. Then I am very poorly and cough for weeks afterwards. I have recently been referred by my GP to a consultant in homoeopathy, and, as a result, I am now on a planned, preventive course of remedies for my susceptibility to infection.

I do not think that there can be a 'cancer personality' (nor ulcer personality, for that matter). I don't feel that I really have much in common with many other cancer patients, except the disease. Considered coldly, I suppose there could be some truth in the idea that cancer can be 'a socially acceptable form of suicide', and I am sure that 'mind over matter' is important for survival.

Looking back these five years since my first primary was diagnosed, although the lump seemed to appear suddenly, I suppose it must have grown very gradually. When I was in hospital, the nurses told me that they were doing their own survey into the causes of cancers: they were sure it was instant coffee drinkers who were the most affected. That didn't apply to me, as I loathe coffee!

If I have to think of a cause, I suppose it could be to do with the family and domestic unhappiness I have had since childhood, especially in my teens and early twenties and at the time of my own marriage, when my parents became quite seriously estranged and there was a great gulf between us.

My father was behaving particularly dreadfully, around this time. Although I was over 21, my fiance had asked permission to marry me. In reply, my father got up and walked out of the room, saying that if that was what we wanted it was up to us, wasn't it? My mother was having serious digestive problems and was in hospital on our wedding day. I felt, in all the circumstances, that I would be happier if my elder brother 'gave me away in marriage', instead of my father. It was a very sad state of affairs and it was only when I walked down the aisle that I noticed that my mother had been quietly brought into church with a nurse. I later learned that they had brought her from hospital in an ambulance.

After that, we didn't see her for 18 months or so. Then, one Sunday morning, as my husband and I were going into the church where we were married, we saw my mother coming out from the earlier service. It was my birthday and she came to our house for tea. But the following ten years were still full of family discord. My father died rather suddenly in 1972, leaving *everything* to my brother. This, of course, had to be contested by my mother and the saga continued bitterly for another five years. My brother kept everything (personal possessions, property, the lot), leaving my mother pretty well penniless. After a hearing at the High Court in London, my brother and his wife were obliged to make a small allowance for my mother. Since then they have completely dissociated themselves from us and have not been seen since!

In the intervening years, I had developed a duodenal ulcer. Also, my husband and I had been going here, there and everywhere for help in trying to start a family. We tried everything, right up to artificial insemination (AIH). Eventually (after we had both had surgery) we decided to adopt, first our son and then our daughter, both right from the 'nest'. We have had medical problems with the boy, but that is another story.

There may well be other causes for my cancers, however, apart from tensions and anxiety. I suspect that hormone imbalance may have played an important part, as I have had very severe mastitis from the time we were married, in 1959. This was possibly the result of having to stifle our desire for children while taking precautions against starting a family too soon from an economic point of view.

I don't think, however, I was ever especially scared of getting cancer myself, as any thoughts about *my* ever having it simply never crossed my mind. I never really thought about it seriously until my mother-in-law died, followed by the deaths of several close friends over the last ten years.

I remember now that my mother had been a patient in the London Homoeopathic Hospital in 1944, for major surgery and successful treatment, post-operatively, with homoeopathy (Calendula,etc.), but I was then only about ten years old and too young to understand the significance of homoeopathy.

My first real introduction to homoeopathy came as a direct result of a TV documentary, in 1979. In this programme a veterinary surgeon spoke of the success in treating animals homoeopathically and on the following day I contacted the Homoeopathic Trust in London. My ten-year-old Labrador dog had been given up by the Surrey Veterinary Hospital, under whose care he had been for some time; they said that nothing more could be done for him. He had become crippled with osteo-arthritis and was practically bed-bound by this time, and we had been given a large bottle of pain-killing tablets and told to increase the dose, as necessary. We were given the option of amputation or euthanasia.

We learned from the Trust that the vet on the TV programme lived in Lindfield, Sussex, and when we phoned him he immediately invited us to bring the dog over to him, from Surrey. He felt that our dog's condition was one he could treat homoeopathically — and this he successfully did in a very short time.

However, just prior to this, fully expecting to have our old dog put down, we had bought a Golden Retriever puppy — to bridge the (proverbial) gap. That was four years ago now and, thus, we have *two* dogs! At 14 years our Labrador recently had a very bad stroke — but, once again, homoeopathy has fully restored him to all his usual activities — and he is still very active indeed!

So it came about that when, a year ago now, my husband and I read that there was to be a lecture on homoeopathy in Haywards Heath, we attended and learned a lot more about the fascinating subject. We immediately became members of the Mid-Sussex Homoeopathic Group, as we wished to support its aims and purposes in promoting understanding of homoeopathy and to encourage preventive medicine and co-operation between allopathic and homoeopathic doctors for the sake of patients.

We were further encouraged when, shortly afterwards, Cancer Contact was formed, and feel that we have derived much moral support from this excellent and well-informed group — and, as a result, much more knowledge about cancer as a whole — its causes and cures. But there is still much to learn.

★

Elizabeth was born in 1929 and is a SRN.

The first symptom I noticed was passing blood per rectum in August 1971 when I was 41. Investigations started at once, but as if there was no urgency. There were stool specimens and a six-week wait for a barium enema. Eventually I was referred to a surgeon who, on rectal examination, found a tumour. Four months had been wasted since reporting the blood in the stools, and I consider I should have been referred to the surgeon earlier. None of the tests are infallible and in my case they all proved negative. During those four months I felt increasingly tired, with intermittent stomach pains low in the abdomen. I had continual morning diarrhoea and ran a temperature: I felt generally unwell, breathless, and shivery with a rapid pulse.

My husband broke the news that I had cancer almost as soon as I came out of the anaesthetic. The operation had been a success, he said; no glands were involved, and I was expected to make a complete recovery. I just didn't want to know, and would have preferred to have been told all this when I was stronger. As I developed intestinal obstruction I had a great deal of pain and ate nothing for 12 days, which I can only compare with 12 days of labour. I then had to have an emergency colostomy. I would not award my surgeon, doctor, nurses and nursing sisters any stars at all. No one mentioned the subject of cancer. My husband was the only person to talk about it, and when he had given me the news, it was never mentioned again.

I can't say I was horrified or terrified by the diagnosis, for when I asked the surgeon if the tumour might be malignant, he had told me 'There is always that possibility'. But I *was* apprehensive. As the operation was, in the end, successful, I had very little reaction from friends and relatives. At no time was I given any advice as to how to prevent future cancers.

Certainly I did want to forget about it all. Apart from the actual cancer, I had a bad time in hospital, especially, I believe, because I was a nurse. If I used correct medical tems, 'the micky was taken', and I felt the staff did not like the fact that I knew as much as I did. To a certain extent I was neglected and left in pain for far too long.

I cannot account for the cause of my cancer. I should by rights have avoided it for I have, most of my life, eaten a diet which is fairly high in fibre and I am very fond of salads, raw vegetables, fruit and wholemeal bread. I did have haemorrhoids when I was 12 but I have always had a good bowel action. I have never smoked, and I drink only a very little alcohol. Maybe we are all predisposed to cancer and we get it in our weakest part. I have never been especially scared of it, and the only member of my family to die of it was my grandfather — and that was stomach cancer — when I was very young. Stress may have been a contributory factor, as I tend to have fairly high standards and am a bit of a perfectionist. Family relationships have been difficult, but curiously enough, were less difficult before I had cancer than they have been since. I tended to shoulder most of the burden of bringing up our two sons, as my husband, who is 16 years older than I am, has not enjoyed good health and has found commuting from Sussex to London exhausting. I felt like a one-parent family!

Recently I have done my own research into cancer prevention, especially with regard to diet, relaxation, yoga and so on. I also joined Cancer Contact. In this mutually supportive group we exchange ideas and findings, which is a great comfort. I no longer want merely to forget about it all, and find it much easier than I did to talk about cancer, especially with other cancer patients. Other patients (including those in the medical profession) are unhappy in such discussions.

The biggest problem, in my opinion, is the lack of information given to patients. Many patients do not know what questions to ask, or how to phrase them. Doctors and consultants seem unable to talk in lay terms, although of course there are exceptions. I have not found being a nurse any help at all! Time is vital: time for discussion. I also think that the 'ward round' is a nerve-racking experience for the patient. Maybe it has to happen, but patients need the opportunity to speak to the consultant alone, in a relaxed manner and atmosphere. I do not think there is any truth in the idea that cancer may be a socially acceptable form of suicide.

★

Veronica was also born in 1929. Neither side of her family had had cancer.

Sudden sharp pains in the breast followed by the discovery of a lump in October 1981 led swiftly to a lumpectomy operation. The morning after, I asked my surgeon if the lump was malignant. He said it was, but was fairly tactful about it. I was horrified, terrified and shocked by the diagnosis.

After the surgery I was given radiotherapy and chemotherapy, but no suggestions about alternative therapies and no advice whatsoever as to how to stay healthy in the future. The attitude was: 'Just go home and forget about it.' I soon realised that this was going to be impossible; I had to come to terms with the fact that I had developed cancer and incorporate it into my experience in some way. I began to realise that I should change my attitude towards certain things: become more philosophical about those I couldn't or hadn't time to do, and try to live one day at a time. I also had to ensure that my general health was as good as it could be. I felt my diet was OK. I have always been careful about taking the right kinds of food, vitamins (especially Vitamin C) and so on, but I am not really faddy; I just believe in being fairly moderate and not eating junk food.

I joined the Mid-Sussex Homoeopathic Group in June 1982 and went to a homoeopathic doctor. Shortly after this I also joined the newly formed Cancer Contact, from which I have derived a great deal of help and support, for instance:

1) Psychological support, talking and writing about what happened to me.
2) Exchanging experience with other members of the group, so that I felt I was perhaps giving, as well as receiving, help.
3) Practical help in selecting and using natural and homoeopathic remedies that contribute to one's general health.
4) Learning relaxation techniques from Lee.

All this is very valuable, especially when one has finished all the conventional NHS treatment and is feeling somewhat alone and isolated in one's experience and uncertain about the future.

I have felt completely at ease discussing cancer with my husband and am fortunate in the fact that my mother, who lives with us, is a most sympathetic listener and is interested in every small detail, so I can 'let off steam' any time I want to. Other people on the whole were kind and concerned, although of course some are nonplussed and don't know how to deal with the subject of cancer.

Why do I feel I got cancer? In my case I feel that

'blood chemistry' had a lot to do with it; cystitis-like symptoms, a breast cyst, and perhaps a general hormone imbalance. I have never been on the contraceptive pill, but I did take Premarin hormone tablets for five years after a total hysterectomy in 1976, which I was given because of fibroids. The hospital told me I would have to take the tablets for the rest of my life. 'You want to stay young and beautiful,' they said! I was never too happy about this, and have raised the subject with a number of doctors over the last few years but never received a satisfactory answer. Two doctors doubted the wisdom of this treatment, especially for women over the age of 50, but two others told me that if I stopped, the menopausal symptoms would be far worse. Only one told me I should make up my own mind about the pros and cons!

When I discovered the lump in my breast my GP told me to stop taking the Premarin immediately. After this another doctor told me that there could be no connection between the drug and the cancer. Yet another doctor in charge of my case said that there was a possible connection, but that no doctor would ever admit it because it was a 'grey area'. I have talked to many women over the last 18 months and am amazed to discover that I know of four living locally who had breast cancer and who had also been taking hormones in one form or another. One of them had an exactly similar experience to mine: hysterectomy, Premarin and then breast cancer. I am suspicious.

Apart from the hormonal imbalance I would admit that I am a tense person who has always had difficulty in relaxing and taking it easy.

I feel that there may be something in the theory of a 'cancer personality'. I am a bit of a perfectionist, which can be wearing; I am always trying to create order in life, which is basically chaotic.

I am an atheist and have always wanted very much to survive. I cannot imagine cancer as a 'socially acceptable form of suicide'. However, I do believe that in some people the will to live and fight can disappear, and that one must be on one's guard against such an attitude. As a feminist I find it ironical that since the age of 40 I have been plagued to my disgust by 'female problems'!

The worst cancer experience for me was the chemotherapy, and the horror that perhaps on any day during the six months of treatment my hair would drop out. It didn't; it only became in poor condition. The feelings of revulsion and nausea were rather horrible, as were the headaches, the hot flushes, the physical exhaustion and a sort of general disorientation.

As far as I was concerned, the National Health Service gave me the works: surgery, radiotherapy, various scans, transport to the hospital, chemotherapy and regular checks. But what is seriously lacking is psychological help, especially in the beginning. The service just isn't geared to this sort of treatment which takes time and money, especially in view of the large number of people involved. What we need is *cancer prevention;* but given the present stage of medical knowledge, is this possible? We are told a pre-cancerous state can exist for 20 years, so ensuring that likely sufferers are screened could be the answer.

I watched the TV series *A Gentle Way with Cancer* with interest. The recommended diet, however, seems formidable. The searching to get organically grown food, spring water, etc. is difficult, time-consuming and tiring at a time when rest and relaxation is needed. It must also have been demoralising to be told you *could* return to orthodox treatment after having munched your way through a lot of raw vegetables. I cannot help feeling that some of the patients on the programme were certainly not average; e.g. two of them said that they were glad they had had cancer, as their lifestyle and attitudes were totally changed. I find this rather masochistic: I cannot ever imagine feeling glad to have had their 'cancer experience' and the traumas that go with it. It doesn't say much for their lives before. One patient took up running (5 miles at a go!) as well as having a nursing job and a family to look after. What enormous energy!

The courage of a woman on the programme who died was fantastic, but I felt I was prying (TV often gives one this feeling) especially when I saw her husband in tears.

The doctor on the programme was rather evasive and non-commital in interviewing patients. The counsellor Penny Bron, on the other hand, was very positive and cheerful except when she said that in the last resort the clinic did help people to die well; this is no small thing. A Glaswegian doctor came across very well with his ideas of treating the whole person and not rejecting anything in the way of conventional treatment.

It was, on the whole, an adventurous series of programmes and it must be good that the BBC gave all this time to discussing an illness which frightens people so much, even if one is not entirely enthusiastic about the Bristol Cancer Help Centre.

★

Judith was born in 1928. There is cancer on both sides of her family. Her husband's family are cancer-free.

My primary breast cancer (in a milk duct) was diagnosed in 1976. A nursing sister told me the news after an exploratory operation following the discovery of a benign cyst. I was very well treated and give ★★★★★ to both my GP and the surgeon who performed the mastectomy operation. My family were all marvellous.

Shortly after leaving hospital I heard about homoeopathic Iscador injections, which a neighbour was having for her own primary breast cancer. I went 'off my own bat' to the homoeopathic hospital and asked for this treatment so as to try to prevent a recurrence of the disease. I have been giving myself these injections ever since. Sometimes I wonder if I am becoming addicted to them, for I feel so much better when I am having them!

I do not dwell on the subject of my cancer, but when one's body has been disfigured one can never forget it. I can discuss anything with anyone, but I don't like being morbid. Everyone has to fight to hang on to life, no matter what.

I think I neglected mastitis after my daughter was born in 1959, and that this may have had something to do with my getting cancer. I breast-fed her, but only for two months and then the milk dried up. I had been well previously, except for a hysterectomy in 1970 for fibroids, and an operation to remove my gall bladder in 1971, but I don't see these as relevant. Perhaps cancer patients do share the same 'body chemistry'.

I don't think I have been more afraid of cancer than I am, say, of a car accident, but I believe very much in Fate.

★

Joanna was born in 1920 when her mother was 40. Her father's side of the family is cancer-free; her mother's cancer-prone.

Since secondary cancer was diagnosed I have been trying to plot a pattern of major traumas or medical events which might be part of the cause. Otherwise I feel sure that a serious shortage of Vitamin C (from a fruit and salad-free diet dictated by a spastic colon), some hormonal imbalance, and an inherited 'organ inferiority' (as Alfred Adler* put it) may have been to blame.

At the age of five I saw Anna Pavlova dance and was

*Dr Alfred Adler (1870-1937) Austrian physician and psychiatrist: founder of the School of Individual Psychology.

bewitched. I had to become a dancer. Shortly after she died in 1931 I had gastric flu and was told that my heart had 'moved'; this makes no sense to anyone now. For a year I was not allowed to dance or play games, but I learned an invaluable lesson from my mother in how to compensate, putting one thing aside only to take up another.

When I was 13 she had a mastectomy, radiotherapy and a lot of pain. My father, brother and I were with her when she died the week before I was 17. The cancer had spread to her lungs, but she was only obviously ill for about two weeks and her death was not at all frightening. In 1938 I had an appendectomy, and during the Munich crisis my father married again, which was best for him but tricky for me. I had made a good start in ballet with Mme Marie Rambert, but when war was declared (and I was in a house that was bombed) I knew that I couldn't dance my way through it. I joined the WRNS, where I soon developed a long-lasting verruca on my foot. My doctor father sent me to a Harley Street man who applied radium and cured it.

Many of my friends were killed in the war and some were especially dear to me. Nevertheless for five years I had the satisfaction of an interesting, responsible job, freedom from domesticity, lots of men and women friends, and good health.

From puberty I had suffered (and I mean suffered) from mastitis. I would be fine (I was told) when I had a baby, but this was something I wanted to avoid until I was married. After demobilisation, at home with my father and stepmother, I had pneumonia and (after being given the new drug M & B) jaundice.

I married in 1948. Most of the next 12 years were spent in Northern Europe enjoying many opportunities and privileges. But my job was now strictly domestic in support of my husband's diplomatic career with its fundamentally anti-feminist and paternalistic lifestyle. I was a perfectionist, and although I found I didn't like cooking, I took immense pains and I cleaned to an absurd degree. It was a lonely life with no demands made on my brain, except for learning four languages ... and I am no linguist. I started writing novels.

During my pregnancy I had no ante-natal care and thought all I had to do was to relax. Our sonwas born in 1949. It was a difficult birth with 'easy' forceps and no one around to speak English or help. Although I couldn't breast-feed our infant for long, my conscience was saved as Stockholm pharmacists sold mother's milk in bottles. He was a very happy baby and child, and although I am not naturally very maternal, my husband and I enjoyed our offspring — all the way.

When he was two my gall bladder plus stones were removed, and a day or so later, a small breast lump. I wasn't at my toughest, and wept because I thought no one would tell me the truth if I had cancer. It was a great relief to be told firmly: 'We don't lie to patients in Sweden.' British doctors often announced that they did, so you couldn't believe them even if the news was good. I had no convalescence and was soon exhausted. A year later I had a duodenal ulcer. I refused to leave my family again, but we were lucky and could afford a good holiday, where I went on a strict diet. The ulcer cleared up. It was about then that we met a woman introduced to us by her son as just having had cancer. From then on I had no difficulty in talking about it.

I was living in England in 1954 when I was rushed into hospital at Xmas with a miscarriage. The nursing sister (refusing to believe that I had an allergy to it) gave me morphia, and was scared by the result. I had a D & C and felt very fit after it. Our son, however, was having a series of feverish colds, proving immune to aspirin and allergic to penicilin. Enough was enough. My mother had been a homoeopath before being converted by my allopathic father, and now my aunt gave me a homoeopathic *Materia Medica* which has proved invaluable. Dr L.R. Twentyman recommended two courses of Iscador injections a year as a cancer preventive. I had them in four countries.

In Denmark when I was 36 a surgeon removed another breast lump. Wearing no masks he and the nurse chatted across my body in Danish as if I couldn't understand. 'If you cut any more away,' said the nurse, 'she'll have nothing left,' and so on. They also didn't believe in my allergy to morphine and I was soon having stomach cramps while the cutting went on above. On the way home we went into a chemist for me to be violently sick. The lump was benign, but I can still hear the knife cutting into my flesh, and I don't like watching TV commercials where chicken breasts are carved!

We were now living in Berlin, where the Army MO wanted to give me hormones for menstrual problems. I refused. When my aunt died of cancer, there were disagreements about her will and I was at loggerheads with those members of my family who had been most dear to me. It was 25 years before I saw some of them again.

We had no choice now but to send our eight-year-old to boarding school in England. This was painful for us all, although the matron at the co-educational Dunhurst was an ideal mother substitute. In 1962, back in Sussex, I was given a partial hysterectomy for fibroids, but no post-operative advice or help. In 1964 two favourite cousins died, one of bowel cancer. Ten days later her husband was found dead in his bed. In 1967 my sister-in-law had a mastectomy and radiotherapy, and a year later, my stepmother had the same operation. In 1969, after I had spent five years writing a book, a publisher — having agreed to publish it — changed his mind. It was a nasty shock for me. I had been having Iscador injections regularly, but now I began to forget to organise them, and virtually stopped.

It was by chance that in October that year a small lump was found in my breast, which needed urgent attention. The surgeon said he would avoid a mastectomy if he possibly could. (Was it irrelevant that he had a beautiful, young wife, I wonder?) I was lucky to be given only a lumpectomy. Hospital, however, is always dicey for patients who want to be treated like adults, especially if they are atheists and refuse to see the chaplain on his intrusive visits! But some of the nurses were really kind. My GP came to tell me that I was to have radiotherapy. I said I had no use for it, even if I did have cancer, which no one had yet confirmed. 'If you want to survive,' he said, 'you have no choice.'

It was on his ward round that the surgeon spent all of half a minute telling me that I had cancer. As he and his troops began to move away, the sister said: 'You can go home now. We need your bed.' I award my surgeon ★★★★★ for his surgery but none at all for his tact. My husband and son deserve a sky-full of stars for their care and loving concern.

Now came decisions. Because of medical prejudices, etiquette and ignorance, my GP would not co-operate with my homoeopathic doctor on my behalf. I decided to have radiotherapy because I felt that if I didn't and then died, my two men might feel I had let them down. I was told that the X-rays would be painless, but that I would burn because of my red hair. In fact, packed around with small 'sandbags' that seemed to weigh a ton on newly scarred tissue, I sweated with pain and could not lie still. After a battle I could have done without, I changed radiotherapists and was given cobalt ray treatment, which was painless. Thanks to my homoeopathic remedies and ointment, I had no burns, but no one at the hospital was interested. I was given no advice as to how to look after myself and it was a Danish friend, a nuclear physicist, who advised me to take strong doses of various vitamins.

Having got used to sleeping drugs in hospital, I was taking two Mandrax every night at home. I was 50 and wasn't going to count myself cured for at least five years, and during that time I had two more scares: a breast cyst and a cyst in my throat. The one was quickly dealt with, the other also harmless. I suffered some black depressions, which my husband found very hard to understand. I believe now this was mostly because of the sleeping pills and radiation. I was given an anti-depressant.

In 1972, my sister-in-law, in the last stages of secondary cancer, took an overdose. It was courageously planned and carried out, as even the coroner agreed. I was already a member of the Voluntary Euthanasia Society and I wished that the law had allowed her a merciful death with medical help, rather than the loneliness and anxiety inevitable in a suicide.

Three years later my blood pressure had reached c.220/140. After five days in a London hospital, I was prescribed Salupres for the rest of my life. This made me more depressed, but other allopathic drugs also had some nasty side effects. My GP was not interested in reporting these. The Committee for the Safety of Medicines said that although few doctors bothered to make such reports, it was no good the patients trying to do anything about it. I read about Dr Bach Flower Remedies, sent for some, and threw away all my orthodox drugs except for one diuretic. My depressions lifted, and homoeopathy continues to control my blood pressure with no problems. I was surprised to realise that in my 'foxhole' I had called on the orthodox medical gods of my father! I was, however, still having Iscador injections regularly, thanks to an arrangement between our homoeopathic doctor and a district nurse. It was many years before I managed to get our GP to prescribe them for me on the NHS.

In 1977 I held our mongrel dog (nearly 18, blind and in arthritic pain) while the vet gave him a lethal injection. I wanted to spare my two men the trauma, but wished I hadn't. While wondering yet again why we are merciful to animals and so unmerciful to human beings, I found that it was all very painful because the body was taken away before I had accepted that the dear animal was dead. Our homoeopathic doctor agreed that the death of a dog or cat can bring as much grief as if they were people.

My husband was due to retire at 60, in May 1979. We had always looked forward to this, but I had realised increasingly that such a change would bring problems for both of us. I wanted to talk about it and make plans: he didn't. Difficulties in communication have been a major cause of stress I couldn't cope with: it wasn't a question of blame, but of different needs and temperaments. Added to this was the fact that only one of the 11 full-length fiction and non-fiction books I had written had been published, although literary agents believed they could sell nine of them. Although I was busy with freelance journalism and many kinds of voluntary work, I had no recognised profession: it all counted as little more than a hobby, and I had virtually no financial independence, even when I started a small postal business in secondhand books.

In April 1979 I began to wake two hours after going to sleep with excruciating pain in my neck and shoulders, which reached my finger tips. I stumbled the night away, moaning. Lack of sleep and exhausted muscles aggravated the problems, which were diagnosed as cervical spondilitis, osteo-arthritis and frozen shoulder. I was prescribed collars, and a splint for my right wrist. I refused traction and had to give up violin lessons. I started instead on the spinet. I took lessons in the Alexander principle, identified some of the causes of the pain, and cranial osteopathy did wonders for me. I even tried acupuncture, but when I got home I found that one of the silver needles had been left sticking into my chest. 'Now that is what I call Chinese take-away,' said a friend. When in 1981 I asked a senior consultant in radiotherapy if radiation might not have dried out my tissues and caused the pain I was having, I was told how lucky I was that radiation had cured my cancer. There were no side effects to worry about. So now I really was cured. I began drastically to cut the dosage and regularity of my Iscador injections. That was one minor discomfort I could avoid.

On retirement my husband had taken over at least half the dreaded meal-getting and he also began to do his own mending. Other women envied me, but my sex has no right to consider men as domestically incapable, often leaving them as helpless widowers. Or so I rationalise my own self-interest. All this meant that my own sphere of usefulness had shrunk. Even the kitchen was not under my control any more. I still had a lot to learn.

I began to lose weight: I lost 13 kg. The pain was now mostly near my cancer scar and going through my back. 'Muscular', said my GP. For some time I had been getting breathless climbing stairs and hills, but, said my GP, so was he. What could we expect at 61? I had to give up playing the recorder. In February 1982 I was rushed to hospital with a suspected perforated ulcer. I was given penicillin (which had no effect). After a gastroscopy, liver scan, and X-rays of my lungs and gall ducts, nothing much was found. There was, however, a neck gland needing a biopsy. I wanted to go home to think about it. My refusal of a general anaesthetic did me no good at all with the surgeon, and the operation was done (after I had waited for many hours, all ready in my theatre gown) by a young doctor. I wasn't sure if he had ever operated before, but he and the nurses could not have been more kind or cheerful.

A week later my husband took me back to hear the diagnosis. A cold, silent nursing sister removed the stitches and said we were to go home again. My husband was to return in two hours. I wasn't invited. I couldn't believe it! Of course we both went back and sat in the queue, saying that we wanted to hear the news together. Then a nurse whisked me away to undress, so the surgeon could look at my neck. It was then that he told my husband, bluntly and with no feeling, that I had secondary cancer. When the surgeon arrived where I lay waiting, suitably submissive on the couch, he gave my neck a cursory glance, and then standing at least six feet above me, told me that I had inoperable, secondary cancers in the lung, breast ... he waved his hand across my body ... 'general disease', with ominous glands also on the other side of my neck. The nurse was running for my husband. 'He wanted to be with her,' she said. He came in, looking very white, but I was beginning to get angry. 'What a way to run a garage,' was my immediate response. I was to take Tamoxifen (an anti-hormone drug) and steroids to make me plump and pink (something I'm not even when I'm well), and have a bone scan. I said that I didn't want the scan, and that I wanted to investigate the drugs before I agreed. 'How long have I got?' I asked. At most two years, possibly three to six months, was the prognosis. The surgeon didn't hang about, and said to my husband as he left: 'If she isn't going to take the drugs, tell her not to get them from the chemist. They are very expensive.' If I could give him fewer than no stars I would. When I told one of our young GPs that I refused to see the man again, he was verging on sympathy, but went on ('as a friend') to warn me to be careful not to upset doctors. I still don't know what we are meant to do when they 'upset' us.

Although in many ways I felt that 62 years were enough, I was determined to prove the surgeon wrong. I immediately started having Iscador injections on alternate days, although my GPs continued to make sure I knew that they regarded them as ineffective faith-healing. Iscador (I was told) worked well with Tamoxifen, so I agreed to that but not to the steroids. I went to a leading herbalist and discovered the value of beetroot and carrot juice and red clover tea. I went to

Gilbert Anderson for visualisation therapy. Our son and his companion gave me an ioniser and encouraged me to continue with T'ai Chi lessons. I went for walks, taking an increasing number of steps per breath. I did wheeze a bit, but homoeopathic Antim Arsenicum stopped that, and Conium dealt with breast pain as it had 12 years ago. I also took homoeopathic Selenium. I realised that wearing nylon had been causing problems, so I stopped, and I gave up eating red meat with its second-hand hormones. There were dozens of books to read, many of which I might not have found if it had not been for our son and friends. I was convinced by now that Vitamin C in large doses would help, and I now take 6 grams a day. Sugar and carbohydrates have always been rather toxic for me: for the first few months I almost cut them out and I took no salt or fat. I learned that cancer patients more often die from starvation than from cancer itself, and if our hospital was anything to go by I wasn't surprised. I had left it with something very close to anorexia, after so many hours starving before tests, and so many meal-times refusing sausages, chips and ice cream. My husband's home-made bread continued to be a favourite basic food. In fact my body began to show signs of a dietary imbalance. It was a long time before I weighed more than 46 kg, and so I began to return to more protein and felt better for it. A homoeopathic nutritionist put me onto enzymes, supplementary minerals and vitamins. It all cost a great deal. If we had not been comfortably off, the surgeon might well have been proved right.

A woman doctor at the Marsden Hospital gave me a second allopathic opinion, with lots of time and patience, confirming my belief that only women doctors can examine breasts painlessly. She, too, wanted bone scans and more X-rays, but again I refused. I have only recently realised that although I could sing moderately well (and high) before being irradiated in 1970, since then I have hardly been able to sing at all. Although my neck scar took some time to go down, and it was suggested that I might need more radiotherapy for that, I was determined to refuse that offer too. It turned out not to be necessary. The swelling subsided.

My own cancers and radiation had increased my concern about nuclear power, tests and weapons, which had to some extent been concerning me in my writing since the 1950s. I now went on the CND marches in London, and felt that with a quarter of a million others, all wasn't totally lost. But there was never enough energy to do everything I wanted to do.

After my first lung X-ray since the diagnosis, my GP phoned and said that, although there had been some regression, there was now some cancer in the ribs. This was the worst news so far, and for 24 hours I felt pretty bad about it. Then I went to the surgery to see the report for myself. He had read it wrong. In fact my lungs were 'clear as a bell' and the regression quite definite. Something had worked, although exactly what I don't know.

Three months after my secondaries were discovered my husband had the first of a series of epileptic fits in his sleep. These were scary, and I was expected to turn his 90 kg onto his side to prevent his tongue from falling back and hampering his breathing, but no one told me that I could wait until the seizure was over (or that there were better ways than butting him with my head). The doctors merely said that I should not call them unless the attack lasted more than 25 minutes. After having to look after me during a long-lasting tummy-bug, the seizures increased in frequency and severity and twice he had two attacks in 24 hours. I began to dread going to sleep and when I dared to try I couldn't. In order to break the cycle, Lee came and nightwatched my husband while I went out of hearing and had a chance to sleep. For this typical act of practical kindness she deserved at least 100 stars. She also taught me how to turn a sleeping man onto his side.

It was seven months before he was given a brain scan and an EEG, both of which were clear. Again our GPs proved less than understanding. Rather than risk 'upsetting' them further, we changed to a local (4-star) homoeopathic GP on the NHS. An SRN told me a story about a man who had secondary cancers and then the most exciting remission. But (she added, not knowing our family history) when his wife developed epilepsy he was so shaken that he was dead in a fortnight! Fortunately, before he was put on large doses of drugs my husband found it very hard to believe that anything had happened to him. A blood, sweat and hair test showed that he was suffering from a poisonous excess of cadmium although no one could give us any idea where this might have come from. The antidote appeared to be zinc. In fact I had given him homoeopathic Zincum Metallicum, the symptoms for which fitted his own quite clearly. After taking a lot more together with other necessary vitamins and supplements the fits began to subside. It had taken more than six months, however, to find the right allopathic drug and dosage; I only wish that people who take one homoeopathic remedy which doesn't work would not conclude that homoeopathy is therefore ineffective!

I have recently had a left frozen shoulder, so neither of us could drive. This time, thanks to the Alexander technique, physiotherapy, cranial osteopathy and T'ai Chi, I am coping much better. The pain varies from a continuous dull 'toothache' type of pain to a sudden 'drilling on an open nerve' if I make the wrong movement; but homoeopathic Hypericum 30 and Chamomilla 3 give me a fairly good night's sleep.

When three years ago I was taking frequent doses of soluble aspirin for the pain, nothing happened, except that I landed up in hospital with a query ulcer. As aspirin is believed to hinder the absorption of Vitamin C, perhaps this was a contributory factor in the development of my secondary cancer.

My 4-star consultant said I should have a cortisone injection. I said 'no thank you'. He said he would book me an appointment. I wrote to him to point out that cortisone and homoeopathic injections do not mix well, and that if homoeopathy was no more than faith-healing, my faith would be severely battered by an injection. I was to have shoulder X-rays, and then after examination, some more, and — if I was 'agreeable' — a bone scan. I again said 'no thanks'. I received notice of an appointment, so I phoned and cancelled it. Until I get symptoms I am not prepared to be subjected to any scanning. My shoulder 'thawed' in six months — a record time. Curiously it was a wasp sting and homoeopathic treatment for it that seemed to accelerate the process.

It is now fourteen years since I had primary cancer which was not cured by surgery or radiotherapy. Homoeopathy may keep it at bay, as long as I keep up the injections. I shall not give them up again. It was in 1962 that I wrote an article about cancer education in the *Guardian* and our local MOH informed me that for women to be better informed about the disease would only lead to widespread cancerphobia. *World Medicine* published my 'Ignorance is Not Bliss' in 1970 and in 1975 my account as a five-year survivor. The BBC *Man Alive* programme asked me to appear on a programme about breast cancer but changed their minds when I wanted to mention homoeopathy and alternative cancer therapies. There has, however, been a marked improvement in the climate of opinion over these 21 years. Several of my elderly friends died in the past, knowing they had cancer but unable to talk to their husbands (who also knew but couldn't admit it). I hope this never happens now. To die with such a lack of trust must be terrible. In 1969 some neighbours drew back as if I were infectious, and a vicar's wife wrote to sympathise and asked me to give her love to a mutual friend who had recently been killed in a car crash! 'Cancer' spelled 'death' to the majority of people, but since 1982 it has been much easier to mention the subject. My husband and son have been wonderful, as have my friends — one of whom phoned Paul Solomon in the USA to see if and when he would be able to give me a healing session in England. Another was going to ask Matthew Manning to give me absent healing, and another produced the Burke book on Vitamin C. Others offered me listening ears, day or night, if I got depressed. Such perceptive kindness was the best therapy of all. Only three friends were nonplussed: one young woman did not reply to my letter for eight months, and then wrote, 'I was a dope giving you up for dead ... I did panic a bit.' Over the last fourteen years, well-meaning Christians (and a Jew) have pointed out from time to time how much I needed a faith like theirs, but my atheist-humanism has served me well, in and out of 'foxholes'.

Cancer Contact has been a splendid source of mutual aid and comfort, and the encouragement, caring and friendships it has produced are invaluable. My biggest problem is exhaustion and getting used to the cancer time-scale, living for today but being aware that if we take 'no thought for the morrow' there may be none for life on this planet.

★

Maura was born in 1916. Her father died of cancer. Her own primary was in the breast.

I had no previous symptoms and didn't notice anything until the lump was visible. The specialist gave me the diagnosis, confirming what I had already suspected. All the same I was absolutely shocked to hear that I had cancer. I was able to talk to my son and daughter and very sympathetic husband. I didn't need help from anyone else and didn't mention the subject.

I was determined not to have a breast amputation unless it was unavoidable, and made this crystal clear to my surgeon when signing the form of 'consent' to the operation. I was very fortunate in that I had instead a lumpectomy. After five weeks of radiotherapy I just put the whole thing out of my mind, like an ostrich digging its head in the sand. No one gave me any advice about preventing a recurrence.

As for the cause: I blame tension and worry and problems with relationships. We had my mother-in-law living with us for six years. And I smoked, but I do not think this is relevant. I think I have always been scared of cancer, but now I feel very much at ease with other cancer patients in Cancer Contact and outside. The worst experience was being told I had the disease. I think it would have helped if I could have talked about it more freely.

Thinking about the various friends who have or have had cancer, I really cannot see any similarity, or believe in a 'cancer type' of personality. One of them smoked until a few years ago: two others never smoked at all. They don't seem to have suffered from stress: one of them is very happy with her husband and job (with no children). Another unmarried friend has enjoyed a very good life and only now, at 78, has to have a lumpectomy. My father, who died of stomach cancer, was very happily married, and was very particular about his food, growing a lot of it himself with no chemical fertilisers, and cooking it correctly. There was stress in his life some 25 years ago, but surely this can't have any relevance after all these years. He was much older than my stepmother.

My Christian faith didn't mean so much to me when I was young, but over the last five years (with other health troubles, including two hip replacements for arthritis), I have found that fear (what is happening?) resentment (why should it happen to me?) and other negative emotions are conquered and I am helped, through my religion, to see things differently.

★

A Nursing Sister's View

This final story is not by a cancer patient, but by the only non-patient member of Cancer Contact, Lee – frequently mentioned above by her fellow-members. Lee was born in 1917. She did her general training at the Liverpool Royal Infirmary and qualified in midwifery at Walton Hospital, Liverpool, and in mental nursing at Chester Mental Hospital, as it was then known.

The next five years, I spent in the Princess Mary's RAF Nursing Service. In 1946 I married. In 1947 my husband, a war casualty, died, and I had to pick up the pieces and go on. I returned to my training school as a ward sister for a further five years, by which time I felt the urge to establish a permanent home. I decided to come south, and these have been for me the most important years of my life.

In Liverpool, cancer patients were always present in my ward. Although my consultants and medical registrars had an extremely humanitarian approach, I felt that there were great limitations on the help that we could give the patients. The orthodox treatment was given without question, and it was considered that the writing was on the wall, and the patients' future very limited. Within the hospital environment I see no improvement today. Outside the hospitals however, I see very great changes. As I have spent more than 40 years in the nursing profession, I feel qualified to make some observations.

We are beginning to recognise the enormous power that our mind exercises over our physical bodies, yet very little attention is paid to this. Everyone will agree that fear is probably the first emotion a patient experiences when told that they have cancer. Fear of pain, of treatment and the appalling side effects; fear of doctors, nurses, of operations; fear of the reaction of husband, wife, children, parents; anxieties about money, of being alone, and of course, fears of dying. Yet I have experienced the crass insensitivity of consultants and doctors when breaking the news to the patient as a bald fact, demonstrating no more than embarrassment and urgency to leave. No attention at all has been paid to these painful emotions which the patient is left to endure in an agony of isolation.

Also it is generally observed that the cancer patient loses weight and appetite. This may be for a variety of reasons, but the hospital diet is very seldom, if ever, geared to help these people when they need a particularly high protein and attractive diet, to replenish the nourishment that the cancer cells devour.

This is a time in patients' lives when they need advice and support, probably more than at any other time. But doctors seldom guide them to ways in which they can help themselves. They frequently pour scorn on the very possibility, failing to recognise that our bodies have a built-in self-healing system of their own, which is remarkably effective when put to use. Patients are left to believe that their treatment has cured them, or that their case is hopeless.

These are well known facts that any cancer patient will confirm. Many people will make excuses for a 'brilliant' surgeon who is 'too busy', and a doctor who really must not be disturbed, when he or she ignores the overwhelming anxieties of the patient and makes it difficult for them to ask questions. How often, for instance, will a consultant sit down quietly and *alone* with a patient, and explain the situation, and then give them hope for their future, allowing them time to question too, expressing a willingness to return if they wish to talk it over? There are of course doctors and consultants who are exceptions, but there are not too many of these.

All my experience was in orthodox medicine until I retired in 1977. It was after this that I met Dr Ainslie Meares, for 30 years a leading psychiatrist in Australia, who has used relaxation with great success in his cancer patients' healing programmes. When I was asked if I would teach this to Cancer Contact I was eager to do so.

When I arrived the house was warm and welcoming. With the exception of one husband and myself, everyone present had cancer. There was one young mother who had very young children, but there were also older women who had made a gallant comeback, after more than one death sentence. The room was bubbling with fun and laughter. Everyone was interested in everyone else. The organiser of the group had a hospital escape record rather like a prisoner whom no gaol can hold. As she led the meeting, the drive that made her live was there for all to see, and she infected others with it.

I played my part as best I could and was both humble and proud to be involved. Let me give you some of my impressions of the group.

I discovered the immense value of each person to the recovery of every other member. Intimate reflections on problems were encouraged, and this resulted in an unloading of many things that had been held tight inside, and members lost their sense of isolation.

I noted that members were all so different from one another, in background environment, intellect and domestic set-up, yet when they joined the group they became important to and loved by every other member.

Cancer Contact did much to eliminate the dreadful fear that I have referred to. Some were more seriously ill than others but they could all talk about their troubles, and because of this their fear tended to evaporate and determination took its place. Each individual seemed to grow in stature in her eagerness to help the others.

I could tell you many individual stories of courage and support. Each member seemed to learn from others in the group. They have open discussion about life and death without any religious barriers. A declared atheist gave a very ill young member a New Testament, believing that it might help. This is the measure of freedom that is important to them all.

Many self-help techniques were made available to the members, who selected the ones that seemed right to them. Nothing was imposed. However, most accepted a measure of diet control; some benefited greatly from the relaxation therapy, while others found it difficult or impossible and preferred to have regular foot massage, known as reflexology. Homoeopathy is widely used within Cancer Contact. Local homoeopathic doctors are an enormous help, and the homoeopathic pharmacist is a tower of strength to all who seek her aid. Most members of Cancer Contact are also members of the Mid-Sussex Homoeopathic Group, although some of them only discovered homoeopathy as a result of having cancer and hearing about it at meetings.

Since becoming involved with Cancer Contact I have learnt so much from the members. This is partly because each is so unique with her own particular needs, and her own special assets. I have learnt too how important constant support is. Not necessarily specialised support, but loving sympathetic support that can accept someone's many changes of mood, even in a day, and help them gently through the despair and depression that most of them experience from time to time. I have watched a young member, going downhill, drag herself out of these dark phases and express gratitude for the few bleak comforts she still had. I observed the pleasure she derived from visits of her friends in the group.

It has always been accepted as important for each member of Cancer Contact to be involved, and though sympathy abounds, courage does too.

No one is allowed to sit and mope. They are all, as it were, in the same boat, and the energy of each one is needed if they are to win and get well again.

The group is growing. In my view groups are needed all over the country, run along the natural therapy and self-help lines. It is the quality of life that is important, and this indeed is where Cancer Contact has helped enormously. It is hoped that there will be an increasing number of doctors, both in hospitals and in the community, who will be open-minded enough to realise that any patient can contribute a great deal to his or her own healing, and advise and direct them to join such a group. I would like to see notices up on every Health Centre notice-board, and in every doctor's quarters, saying 'Nearest Cancer Contact'. After all, who is to know which of us will need it next?

III. Therapies Old and New

1. Detection and Prevention

Many of the cancer organisations produce their own information booklets, and they list the major signals to look out for when it comes to cancer:

1) Unusual bleeding or discharge.
2) A lump or thickening of the breast or elsewhere.
3) A sore that does not heal.
4) Persistent changes in bowel or bladder habits.
5) Persistent hoarseness or cough.
6) Persistent indigestion or difficulty with swallowing.
7) Any changes in a wart or mole.

There is also recent evidence to show that genital warts (three times as common as herpes) can cause cancer of the cervix, from which 2,000 women die every year, some of them very young. Inevitably it is women's sex-life that is blamed and strong indications of other risk factors are ignored. These include, of course, male sexual behaviour, carcinogenic sperm in some men, smoking, vitamin deficiencies, occupational hazards, and some oral contraceptives. Little propaganda is seen in Britain about sexual hygiene. Bidets are still thought of as 'foreign' or imagined to be designed for washing feet. Schools are notoriously slack in teaching basic cleanliness, which may nevertheless be a luxury for many adults living in slum conditions with one bathroom shared among many families. Screening against cervical cancer places women in a passive role. Since so many women's organisations contribute generously to cancer research, it is time they asked how their money is being spent.

We are discouraged from examining and touching our own bodies, and women may be especially inhibited about this. It is easier to believe that you have no symptoms than to go to a doctor (and most doctors are still male) and be examined in parts of your body which you have not seen yourself! Virgins may refuse even to contemplate smear tests, whereas a woman doctor in a Well Woman Clinic could put their minds at rest. Some of the most important reforms in health care have been instigated by the Women's Movement, and understanding and enlightenment grow as women talk more openly with one another.

Some people are afraid of reporting suspicious symptoms for fear of being accused of cancerphobia; but it is much better to be unfairly labelled 'neurotic' or even a 'trouble-maker' in a good cause (and what better than your health?) than to become seriously neurotic from stifled anxiety and be forced to make trouble in order to get the treatment you want. The taboo that still clings to the word 'cancer' breeds fear, and fear is the most common cause of neglecting cancers in the early stages. The more we talk about cancer as freely as we talk about other ailments (especially if we have it ourselves) the better. In the experience of Cancer Contact, men find it especially hard to discuss the problems.

When you have reported your symptoms there are many methods used for diagnosis, from cervical smear tests and screening to manual examinations, ultrasonic or X-ray scanning. You are of course allowed to have a second opinion, although things can move so fast once danger signs have been detected that it may take a lot of concentration to arrange. Generally, orthodox practitioners will admit to there being mistakes in diagnosis only when what they have said was cancer disappears thanks to some alternative treatment!

If you are tempted to rely on an unorthodox healer's intuition for a *diagnosis,* it is as well to double-check with someone who is medically qualified.

There is increasing evidence that the cancer-prone

have abnormalities in their hormone levels and that these can be detected many years before the disease is diagnosed. This was reported in 1976 (*Sunday Times* June 13th). In April 1983 the Imperial Cancer Research Fund suggested that cancer of the breast and ovaries might be prevented by identifying women with hormone imbalance as much as ten years before diagnosis by other means, and by a simple blood and urine test. It must surely be possible by now to carry out these tests on a regular basis. There is never any shortage of money, as we know, when it comes to 'defending the country' with cancer-producing nuclear weapons.

In 1979 it was reported that some Indian doctors were claiming that mental and heart disease could be diagnosed by studying a patient's fingerprints, and doctors at the Amritsar Medical College in the Punjab stated that fingerprints of patients with cancer of the breast, uterus or blood also showed deviations (*Guardian* June 12th 1979). Members of Cancer Contact, with the help of a friendly policeman in CID and an Indian doctor friend, are making their own investigations.

Cancer, as we know, is not one disease but hundreds, and their causes are still shrouded in uncertainties. Although cancer is not strictly hereditary, we may inherit what Alfred Adler (the Austrian psychologist) labelled an 'organ inferiority' which leaves us especially at risk in that particular area.

Within the last few years there have been a number of 'breakthroughs'. Two groups from the USA led by Dr Robert Weinberg and Dr Mariano Barbacid discovered how a gene turns a normal cell into a cancer cell. They found that a single nucleotide (building block) of the DNA that makes up the gene is replaced by another, the cancerous gene in turn manufacturing a protein called P21 (which is only one amino acid different from the innocent variety). That difference is enough to produce a cancer cell (*Guardian* November 12th 1982). In July 1983 at the Imperial Cancer Research

Fund laboratories in London a computer expert, Peter Stockwell, found a close resemblance between a substance in human blood called PDGF and the virus that causes cancer in monkeys. PDGF is a clotting agent which heals cells around a wound, but this can be switched on by a chance mutation (caused by a carcinogen like radiation or cigarette smoke) and go into action when it shouldn't; a cell divides, and tumours are rapidly formed. It was stated that the drug companies would soon be producing new biological drugs which 'will make the present generation of cancer drugs look extremely harsh' (*Sunday Times* July 10th 1983). But there are bound to be problems when interfering with the body's natural healing mechanisms, so we go from 'breakthrough' to 'breakthrough' and (for all the millions of pounds and dollars spent on orthodox cancer research) we still don't know why one quarter of the populations of western societies will get cancer and why the other three-quarters will not. It is this that we urgently need to know. Why, for instance, do sharks so rarely develop cancers, and what is it about basking-shark cartilage extract that blocks the growth of tumours? The alternative oncologists can hardly be considered less successful than their orthodox colleagues, and if they had only half as much money to spend on research, who knows what might not be achieved?

A large part of the story of cancer is guesswork, and often bad guesses at that. There are countless contradictory reports about what is and what is not carcinogenic (cancer producing): one year a product is denounced as potentially lethal and the next it is said to be safe or even good for you. Perhaps all substances should be considered neutral and the emphasis placed more on the processing before and after they enter our bodies. Some substances like radium, plutonium, uranium, asbestos and nicotine tar are dangerous for most people, but even so some people will be able to produce enough defence mechanisms to prevent cancers from forming. What matters is dosage, the amount the body absorbs and the extraordinarily complicated balance in the body of friends and foes, nutrients and toxins.

Governments prove they are worried even when insisting that the steps they are taking are perfectly safe. Uranium is being mined well away from people governments think 'matter'. Thus in the USA one quarter of the world's deposits of uranium come from the once beautiful Indian reservations, while in Namibia it is only black Africans who have to work the mines. Nearly half Britain's uranium comes from Namibia, and so we did not even protest when 60,000 South African troops invaded the country in order to ensure our supplies of the deadly metal. Those who have dared to question the safety of our nuclear power programme, such as Dr John Gofman and Dr Thomas Mancuso in the USA, have had their contracts terminated. In September 1982 in Britain, Dr Rodney Fordham of the UK Atomic Energy Authority was forced into early retirement for questioning the official position on pressure vessel safety in the Pressurised Water Reactor, and Dr Hesketh was sacked for questioning the nuclear authorities.

John Gofman (discoverer of Uranium 233) wrote: 'The majority of scientists had the same stupid attitude as I did ... that if there are any problems, we scientists can fix everything if you give us enough money. And that, if you don't know the effects of low-level radiation, you don't stand in the way of progress; you go ahead. And there are scientists today who say that. Of course today we know about it, so they're even worse than experimenting on humans; they're murdering humans' (quoted in *Guardian* November 29th 1983).

Immunology:

Only one in three people deliberately infected with cold virus actually catches a cold, and we don't know why. We can land on the moon, or destroy our planet at the touch of a button prompted by a faulty computer or a flock of geese, but we still know very little about the science of immunology. The new epidemic disease causing sickness and death, especially in the USA, is known as AIDS which stands for 'acquired immune deficiency syndrome', and clearly a far better understanding of this 'deficiency' is needed. Lucien Israel's book *Conquering Cancer* [30] is a good introduction to the subject of immunology. He writes:

> 'On the basis of a considerable number of convergent studies, we can now state that the blood of some persons who have tumours contains certain substances that block the specific immunity to tumour cells and others that, in a non-specific way, block all the immune mechanisms. In other words, tumours manufacture ... or cause the organism to manufacture (as I myself and many others have shown) substances that protect them from immunologic aggression' (p.154).

So our defence system has to be more powerful than that of the tumour.

Israel goes on: 'Immunotherapy, then, is the youngest brainchild of medical oncology. It seems to be of sound constitution and promising development. But it still requires close supervision' (p.156). It is a pity that he doesn't mention homoeopathy or its possible beneficial effect on the immune system, especially with the Iscador remedy used against cancer.

We are clearly still stumbling in the dark when it comes to cancer prevention, and too many questions are not being asked. How do our own immune mechanisms differ from those of the tumour? If we stimulate one, do we necessarily stimulate the other? Surely we can find substances that are lethal to even the best-defended cancer cells but leave the healthy undamaged? How do vitamins and Laetrile stand up under this sort of investigation? How can patients get blood tests to show how well their immune systems are faring under stress, other diseases, and so on?

There is said to be a latent period of 20 years between exposure to what the individual body recognises as carcinogenic and the development of the disease. This is both good and bad. Nearly 40 years after we dropped atomic bombs on Japan, people are still dying there as a result of radiation-induced cancers, as are men who were involved in the testing of nuclear bombs since the war. Nevertheless, although 1,000 metres from the hypocentre of the Hiroshima bomb there was a 50 per cent increase in leukemia, not everyone who survived got cancer. Or they may have had it and it was defeated by their immune system. Our body cells are regularly renewed (except for those in our brain), so we are continuously being given opportunities to overcome the risks we have run. We dare not waste these opportunities.

Professor Richard Doll, honorary director of the Imperial Cancer Research Fund and Clinical Trials Unit, Britain's leading medical statistician, has said that 80-90 per cent of cancers are preventable. He and Dr Richard Peto, the ICRF reader in cancer studies, were asked by the American government to prepare a report on the avoidable risks of cancer in the USA today. They found that the largest single factor causing cancer was diet: 35 per cent (38 per cent if alcohol is included in the diet). The second most important factor was tobacco at 30 per cent. None of the 'also-rans' came above 10 per cent. Wisely, Doll and Peto avoided the quicksands of speculation about 'psychological causes' which they merely listed under 'unknown causes'. It is a pity more oncologists do not follow their example.

To sum up: Most of us accept that early detection is a good way of preventing the development of cancers already *in situ,* and if it is true that our bodies are creating and destroying cancer cells all the time then this preventive measure may be enough, so long as it is not only local symptoms that are treated. The fact remains, however, that some early treatment is drastic and the cancers might have resolved themselves if left alone. It has been concluded that mass X-ray screening for breast cancer resulted in approximately 5 per cent more cancers than were detected,* and so the discussion 'to screen or not to screen' continues. There is a lot of medical faith in early detection, but it is not necessarily life-saving and this must partly be because cancer is not yet recognised as a constitutional disease, or rather that it is many different diseases all affecting the whole person. We need to take the searchlight away from local symptoms and provide efficiency tests for immune systems. Everything that threatens those defences should be listed as enthusiastically as are carcinogens today.

Cancer Contact discussed 'scans'. Some of us felt that when there are no symptoms we are justified in refusing tests which are of academic interest to doctors only (especially if the patient has already been proclaimed 'terminal', and 'inoperable'). Where there *are* symptoms, however, that is a very different matter, especially if they give pain or cause any anxiety at all. As soon as we have a diagnosis we can see what can be done, homoeopathically or by alternative therapies. There may well be time enough to get rid of the cyst before the doctors want to see it again for re-measuring. And by doing something, worries are relieved. There are many definitions of the 'optimist': in our terms the person who is properly optimistic is the one who recognises that although one in ten breast

**Radiation: The Facts They Don't Want You To Know,* from Nuclear Information, P O Box 11, Godalming, Surrey.

lumps may be cancerous, this means that nine out of ten are harmless. Even when we find we have danger signals in our body, that body has strong healing powers which can be put to good use by the 'gentle methods' of cancer prevention and care.

2. The Orthodox Options

The basic orthodox methods of treatment for cancer are surgery, radiotherapy and chemotherapy.

Surgery may be necessary if the tumour is obstructing vital organs.

Mastectomies have long been considered the only possible means of dealing with breast cancer, and although our bosom-obsessed society suggests that breasts are essential if women are to function successfully sexually and domestically (and especially in advertising promoting the sale of almost anything) women who have one or two breasts amputated are not considered 'disabled'. Perhaps some of the guilt some cancer patients feel about getting the disease is not entirely unrelated to the fact that women who are victims of assault, from the grievous bodily harm of rape to wife-battering, are often treated as guilty rather than as the victims they are. Mercifully, as far as cancer is concerned, amputation is no longer accepted as the only useful operation, and 'lumpectomies' (removal of the tumour but not the whole breast) are good news. It is also good that women have begun to value themselves as people rather than as 'vital statistics', and perhaps it will not be too long before the one-breasted or even the no-breasted can feel as self-confident topless as their top-full sisters. Horrific reports that in America some women are asking for their breasts to be amputated as a means of preventing cancer demonstrate how little cancer is recognised as a constitutional disease. For women who are not able to avoid a mastectomy and are seriously unhappy about their lack of curves, there are encouraging results from various forms of plastic surgery, as one member of Cancer Contact was able to describe. These too, however, have side effects that should be understood.

Radiotherapy: Cancer cells can be destroyed by the use of strictly localised exposure to X-rays or gamma rays, or the radiant energy of radioactive sources such as radium or cobalt 60. There is also new equipment, the linear accelerator, which treats cancerous tissue by penetrating it with high-energy radioactive beams. Such treatment shrinks tumours. Unfortunately it also shrinks and throws into imbalance other body tissues.

Side effects of radiotherapy depend on the concentration of the dose, the site of the treatment and the idiosyncrasies of the patient; they may range from nausea, sickness and depression to muscular pain many years after treatment. Fair skins are liable to burn, but homoeopathic remedies can be extremely effective and may prevent burns altogether. Itching is another problem, for which orthodox doctors often prescribe cortisone-type lotions.

There is continued discussion as to what is and what is not a 'safe dose' of radiation, taking into consideration the existence of the risks we cannot avoid from the environment, television screens and so on. All we can say is that there is no longer any level at all which we can be sure really is safe, and the best we can do is to have as little as possible. It is interesting to note that 'pills to protect the people from radiation' caused by an accident at a nuclear power plant, the dumping of nuclear waste at sea, or war, are being stockpiled in the Isle of Man. These pills contain potassium iodate, which makes glands resistant to cancer (*Guardian* June 13th 1983). Very rarely, however, do we hear of any patient receiving radiotherapy treatment who is given any advice as to how to counteract the side effects. Indeed, few people are given the opportunity to discuss what is to be done, or hear about any alternatives, before they are involved in the hospital routine. If people are interested and want to know what is being done to them, they should not hesitate long before asking a lot of questions: things can happen very quickly once cancer has been diagnosed.

The immune system inevitably suffers from radiotherapy, which depletes the body's supply of vitamins and minerals which it is essential to replace. Anything that kills cancer cells will also kill healthy cells, and this fact must not be forgotten.

In 1976 Dr Donald Gould wrote an article 'Cancer — A Conspiracy of Silence' (*New Scientist* December 2nd 1976). In this he quoted an American scientist who was asked why all 'the enormous amount of money and effort which have been squandered (it is hardly too strong a term) upon the cancer problem over the past several decades have so far resulted in almost no benefit at all for the cancer sufferer'. One of the scientists he spoke to replied: 'It just doesn't serve to rock the boat ... Look, when you've got ten thousand radiologists and millions of dollars worth of equipment, you give radiation treatment even if study after study shows that a lot of it does more harm than good.'

As Dr Gould went on to say, a small but significant number of patients 'can be relieved of distressing and disabling symptoms, and can be given extra months or years of useful and enjoyable life, by surgeons, radiotherapists and physicians skilled in the handling of the disease'. This is, he says, wholly commendable. To warn people of the dangers might be to dissuade them from reporting early symptoms. The orthodox oncologists have then created their own Catch 22: the least they can do is to break 'the conspiracy of silence' and to recognise the very real value of alternative therapies in order to minimise the failures of orthodoxy.

Headlines like 'I Will Die For My Unborn Baby' (*Sunday People* August 7th 1983), the story of a 'tragic mother-to-be' who offered to sacrifice her own life to save her unborn child by refusing radiotherapy treatment for cancer of the liver which was discovered during a routine pregnancy check, ought to be banned by the Press Council. Mrs Sheryl Skirton had been told that 'the only hope of prolonging her life was immediate radiotherapy'. Or perhaps it is the medicos who told her that who ought to be struck off. There is never one 'only hope': it is dishonest and psychologically destructive to suggest that there is.

Chemotherapy is the use of drugs to kill cancer cells. These can be especially useful in the treatment of children with leukemia and people with advanced Hodgkins' Disease. As the drugs are extremely toxic (one of them is related to mustard gas) it is important to compensate for this as much as possible. (See Sections 5 & 6 below.) There is the story of a man whose 'extreme toxicity' saved his life, but in an unusual way: he was a drug addict in India who was bitten by a poisonous snake and survived. The snake, however, died. There must be a moral in this somewhere, if only for zoo keepers on chemotherapy!

Some of the orthodox drugs given to cancer patients kill and weaken the hair passing through the hair follicles, so that when the hair appears it breaks off. Although it grows again, many people would rather avoid this 'side effect'. At the Royal Marsden Hospital there are experiments being carried out to see if the hair can be saved by 'freezing' the patient's head. It takes a brave woman or man to endure some of the attempts to cure cancer, and Ingrid Bergman told a friend of Cancer Contact that as far as she was concerned the treatments during her last illness were worse than the disease.

The choice for cancer patients will often be between living longer or making life worth living. It is alarming to read that drug trials are carried out on patients without their approval or even knowledge. The British Medical Association justifies this by saying that these patients cannot be told they have cancer; either they do not want to know or their doctors believe that they could not bear being told (*Here's Health* June 1982). This shows that there is all the more reason for widespread propaganda to help people face the facts of cancer, as they are able to face so many other problems that beset them.

One of the problems, however, is that even those people who are quite prepared to face the truth are not being told it. James Dewey Watson (1962 Nobel prizewinner for medicine) has called America's cancer programme 'a total sham' [43]. Dr Watson told a symposium on cancer research at the Massachusetts Institute of Technology: 'The American public is being sold a nasty bill of goods about cancer. While they're being told about cancer cures, the cure rate has improved only about 1 per cent.'

Dean Burke of the American National Cancer Institute has protested that in the screening programme to discover new cancer-killing materials at the Cancer Chemotherapy National Service Centre, 'Ascorbic acid has been bypassed, excluded from consideration and never tested for its cancer killing properties'. The reason given was that ascorbic acid is too non-toxic to fit into the research programme! ([43] p.92).

Professor M.D. Rawlins of the Clinical Pharmacology Department at the University of Newcastle-upon-Tyne, wrote to the *Guardian* (April

5th 1983): 'The notion that serious illnesses require strong medicine with unpleasant side effects is so widely accepted that Mrs Thatcher herself uses the analogy in defence of her economic strategy! What does disturb people is the knowledge that drugs used for symptomatic relief, for disorders that get better on their own, or for preventive purposes, may kill or maim as many as one in ten thousand of those who take them.' As he went on to say, an airline or car industry that killed that number of people would soon go out of business. The professor believes that what we must do is to manoeuvre the profit motive to our own advantage and push the pharmaceutical industry in the direction of service to society as a whole, rather than the demands of its shareholders. Who is brave enough openly to disagree with that?

Communication: a major failure in the training at medical schools is the art of communication. Doctors and surgeons who may be experts in their specific practical skills can be walking disasters when it comes to communicating with their patients, and probably cause as much stress as some will suffer in a lifetime. A ward sister wrote that training is 'all anatomy and physiology, how to deal with a gall bladder rather than a person. It's a disgrace ... communication counselling should be in the very first part of the training' (*Guardian* June 29th 1983).

It takes very little time indeed to show genuine concern for a person facing the future with cancer: until everyone in the medical profession learns to offer support without orders, information without dogmas, and co-operation with interest, the rest of hospital care may count for nothing. Medicos with personality problems would do well to experiment on themselves with homoeopathy and Dr Bach remedies.

3. Homoeopathy

Dr Samuel Hahnemann (1755-1843), a German physician, was dissatisfied with his profession. He wrote: 'I conceive that medicine, although apparently highly scientific in its theories, is in practice little more than an empirical and routine application of remedial measures, of which we know neither the certain effects nor the laws which should determine their choice. I shall no longer remain connected with an art which both my understanding and my conscience condemn as insufficient and injurious.' In 1790 he translated the Scottish doctor Cullen's *Materia Medica*, and was attracted by a reference to bark and its seemingly incompatible properties. He was fit and well and he decided to take large repeated doses of bark, whereupon he developed febrile symptoms very like those of ague or malaria, for which cinchona bark was believed to be a specific cure. Hahnemann went on to experiment on himself (and later on his family) with other medicines reputed to be specific for particular diseases. Like Albrecht von Haller (the 'founder of modern physiology') he stressed the importance of testing drugs on healthy people. In patients who were ill you could never be sure which symptoms were caused by the disease and which by the remedies taken for it. Many of the substances he and his colleagues tested were poisonous, and their symptoms were carefully noted. When patients suffering similar symptoms were given small doses of the same substance, it was found that they were effectively cured.

After long and painstaking research Hahnemann concluded that: 'Diseases are cured by such medicines as have the power of producing in the healthy organism symptoms similar to those which characterise the disease itself.' The homoeopathic maxim was born:

'Similia similibus curentur' or 'Like cures like'. His first publication in 1805 resulted in bitter opposition, both from his orthodox colleagues and from the pharmacists, and he and his family suffered considerably for his 'heretical' ideas. He was however an uncomfortable zealot to work with.

The homoeopathic 'minimum dose' evolved slowly as the system developed, and it provided the critics with even more material for ridicule. Nevertheless Hahnemann was able to write: 'Every medical man who adopts homoeopathy distrusts these small doses, till experience proves to him their particular adaptation for the cure of the disease.' The fact is that if a person is given a quantity of plain mercury or quicksilver, it will merely pass through the stomach and bowel and be voided without having any effect. If however the mercury has been very finely divided by grinding for a long time with some chalk, thus producing what is known as grey powder, it will act as an aperient when taken.

Dr Hahnemann believed that our bodies have a natural ability to heal themselves, and that his remedies could stimulate that healing power, whereas orthodox medicine all too often suppressed it. Homoeopaths have always set out to treat the patient as a whole individual rather than as a collection of unrelated symptoms, and the remedies are prescribed to treat the whole person rather than isolated parts of the body. Apart from local injuries, said the homoeopaths, all diseases affect the whole person. Hahnemann was also ahead of his time (and not all his followers agreed with him) in believing that chronic diseases were caused by chronic conditions, like bad housing, polluted water, or too little fresh air and exercise; in such cases more was needed than homoeopathic remedies.

The anonymous author of *A Concise View of Homoeopathy* wrote: 'The cure of chronic diseases is as precarious today as it was a century ago ... Would it not be natural to suppose that any real progress in practical medicine would be hailed with joy by those engaged in its exercise; and that any discovery holding out even a distant hope of improvement would induce an eager, candid and experimental examination? That this, however, is not always the case, the history of homoeopathy sufficiently proves.' That was written in 1848. Although homoeopathy has been part of the National Health Service since its inception, the 'hailing with joy' is still only a whisper. The prejudices that Hahnemann suffered from die hard.

Homoeopathy today is more widely respected in Europe and Asia than in Britain, where it is not taught in our medical schools. As a result the orthodox medical hierarchy refuses to recognise it as a post-graduate subject, which means that doctors cannot get grants for the extra training they need in order to qualify in homoeopathic medicine. The survival of the homoeopathic hospitals is constantly threatened, and thousands of patients are deprived of the homoepathic treatment they want and which is their due. In July 1983, however, the *British Medical Journal* published an interesting report on alternative medicine showing that out of 86 general practitioner trainees, 70 wanted training in homoeopathy and other alternative techniques (*BMJ* July 30th 1983).

Homoeopathic remedies are safer and cheaper than orthodox (allopathic) drugs, but homoeopaths do not deny the value of allopathy or surgery in certain cases. If the NHS is serious in wanting to save money and to get its priorities right, the first step should perhaps be to make full use of homoeopathy, not least as preventive medicine.

Members of Cancer Contact who had been using specific homoeopathic treatment for the disease (see Iscador) were excellent advertisements for the system, and many people joined the Mid-Sussex Homoeopathic Group because they saw the results. One CC member walked into a plate-glass window: she had no concussion but a severe headache and stars. She had with her (and used) homoeopathic Accident Pills, Arnica Cream and Dr Bach Rescue Remedy, and suffered no bruising; the headache went, and by the next day it was impossible to convince anyone of what had happened.

Homoeopathy is invaluable for treating infants and animals, and cannot therefore be described as faith-healing, its remedies no more than placebos. So far, however, there is no easy explanation as to how and why it works; new discoveries in physics may provide some of the answers. We are getting used to thinking of the universe and its stars and planets as being so many light-years away: we have to get used to the idea of the power of substances in minute, even sub-atomic doses, for as homoeopaths know, these can have a powerful healing effect.

The Homoeopathic Handbook (published annually by A. Nelson and Co. Ltd, 73 Duke Street, Grovenor Square, London W1M 6BY) provides a good introduction to homoeopathy, with lists of doctors who are members of the Faculty of Homoeopathy (M.F. Hom.) and chemists who sell homoeopathic medicines. Information is also available from the Homoeopathic Development Foundation, Harcourt House, 19a Cavendish Street, London W1M 9AD, and Ainsworths (Homoeopathic Pharmacy), 38 New Cavendish Street, London W1M 7LH (tel. 01-935-5330) supply remedies, book lists and simple *Materia Medica* for domestic use. Beginners should always ask for information about dosages and the care of remedies.

Dr Bach Flower Remedies: Dr Edward Bach (1886-1936) was a Harley Street physician who was converted to homoeopathy and then went on to develop his own remedies from flowers. Whereas homoeopathy treats both the physical and the mental, Dr Bach believed that physical problems are caused by our emotional states. Accepting 'I don't feel myself today' as a sign of sickness, he aimed to help his patients feel 'more like themselves' rather than to conform to some imaginary norm. Dr Bach's drops are effective in relieving stress, from grief and depression to terror and panic: they correct any imbalance so that we can live at ease with life. As Nickie Murray (of the Bach Centre) writes: 'The thing about drugs is that they don't allow us to battle with life any more, to find our own resources, make decisions. We become like cabbages. It's so sad ...'

One Cancer Contact member had received a poison pen letter, and on reading it felt faint, sick and ill. She had just got some of the Dr Bach Rescue Remedy, and she took five doses at ten minute intervals. After an hour she felt completely composed, and quite determined to take every possible practical step to make sure no one else received similar mail.

Bach remedies are relatively inexpensive, anyone can prepare their own; they are completely safe, can be taken even when we are on orthodox drugs, and work equally well for infants and animals. Some people also use them for plants and trees.

The first problem for most cancer patients is to learn how to live with the diagnosis; some anxiety and depression are almost inevitable. Dr Bach's remedies may make it unnecessary for a person to take allopathic tranquilisers or sleeping drugs, but even if they don't, they help. The best testimonial usually comes from relatives: 'she's much happier' or 'he's much easier to live with' and that can't be bad. [13 & 58] Write to the Dr E. Bach Centre, Mount Vernon, Sotwell, Wallingford, Oxon, OX10 0PZ.

Iscador: It was Rudolf Steiner who saw a connection between cancer and mistletoe, both of them being parasites absorbing the 'life forces' of the parent body. He first produced Iscador (fermented viscum album) in 1933, and research continues to this day. In *Clinical Experience with the Mistletoe Preparation 'Iscador'* Rita Leroi writes: 'It has been experimentally established that the mistletoe in therapeutic doses brings about a stimulation of the thymus, the central organ of the cellular immune reaction. These, and other experiments, e.g. the stimulation of phagocytosis, the increase of immune-competent lymphocytes after the clinical application of Iscador, the proliferation of granulocytes, show that the mistletoe also works on the other pole of the cancer process, namely the immunological surveillance, which is the expression of the individual form-giving and form-maintaining forces of organisation.' She also states: 'It is striking that Iscador leads to a highly significant improvement of the survival quota in those prognostically unfavourable cases with lymph node involvement,' and as regards breast cancer: 'Without post-operative irradiation and without hormonal interference, all patients who have undergone partial resection have a better life expectancy, which in the first three years is statistically significant.'

Cancer is, Rita Leroi reminds her readers, a failure of the immune system within an environment beset with carcinogenic influences. 'A true cancer therapy requires the engagement of the total human capacities of the doctor who, despite setbacks, should not allow himself to become discouraged in his struggles with the disease. The doctor should win the patient as a partner in this fight. Or, to put it another way: while orthodox cancer treatments are used to destroy the cancer cells, Iscador therapy is directed not only at the malignancy but at restoring the equilibrium between organism and cell, by stimulating the form-giving processes of the whole organism.' We also read in 'Directions for the Use of Iscador' that 'harmful effects have not been reported' (and that was after 47 years); 'Iscador therapy given concurrently with irradiation will improve the patient's tolerance of radiotherapy.'

The Anthroposophists (followers of Rudolf Steiner) have a philosophy that is not for everyone, but on this account to reject out of hand what they have to offer in homoeopathic treatment is to mock the cancer patient. Steiner was one of the first ecologists, warning us in the 1930s of world food shortages as a result of soil sickness and over-production. Diet is included in the Steiner therapy today, and it is refreshing to read: 'One should never be too dogmatic. Often a bit of meat added to the diet, an egg, a little chicken, or even a soused herring will be better than vegetables eaten with distaste.'

4. Complementary Medicine and Therapies

Homoeopathy is not included in this section because it is an intrinsic if neglected part of the National Health Service.

Thomas Carlyle wrote about 'the difference between Orthodoxy or My-doxy and Heterodoxy or Thy-doxy'; the dividing line between 'quackery' and the established medical practices shifts, and is often hard to detect. When people were forbidden to interfere with what was considered the monopoly of God the Great Healer, scientists concentrated on making weapons of destruction and war. The only acceptable and legal therapy was prayer for the cure of the soul, and in more serious cases, exorcism to drive out the devils of disease. The 'alternative therapists', the women and the wise men with their herbs, potions and charms, risked being burned alive as witches in their attempts to ease suffering.

The ancient sciences and medical knowledge remained in the hands and lands of the Arabs, who were 'heretics', as were the Jews, who forged the link between the Pagan Light and the Dark Ages of Faith, bringing with them the forgotten knowledge of medicine and helping to found our earliest medical schools. They were also pioneers in the field of public health and laid great stress on personal hygiene in what was a very grubby time.

In the Middle Ages, Valentine Schindler, the German scholar, wrote: 'Physicians do not discover and learn everything they ought to know in the universities; they often have to go to old wives, gypsies, masters of the black art, old peasant folk, and learn from them. *For these people have more knowledge of such things than all the colleges and universities.*' [37]

Increasingly, 'drugs' meant 'poisons' for which the druggists charged exorbitant prices, thus preventing efforts to reduce the cost of medical treatment. Gradually the belief that disease was punishment from God faded, although it has not entirely vanished today. The clashes between theology and science, magic and medicine, orthodoxy and heresy continued, and the scope for charlatanism on the one hand and injustice on the other was so great and exploited so widely that it is no wonder the public is still bemused.

Even inside the medical establishment life was not easy for the pioneers and innovators. Their theories about smallpox vaccination (brought from Turkey by Lady Mary Wortley some 80 years before Edward Jenner faced the scorn of his colleagues), anaesthetics and antiseptics were denounced as blasphemy. The fully qualified physicians who were also homoeopaths were the target for attack not only by the pharmacists: in 1851 the Medical Society of London decreed that its members could not honourably hold professional communion with them. Official medicine continued to be dangerous, with its blood-lettings and poisons in lethal doses. 'Orthodox' was no guarantee of safety: it was merely respectable.

In the mid 19th and early 20th century there were two 'famous' treatments for cancer: the Hoxsey Cancer Formula and Dr Coley's fluid. Both were damned outright as quack and added to the blacklist of unproven cancer treatments. In the late 1970s, however, evidence of a survival rate among patients diagnosed as terminal brought these theories into a much more favourable light. Dr Coley had used a preparation of heat-killed bacteria which induced fevers and chills. Today some orthodox doctors are experimenting with heat therapy: Dr Donald Cole of the Holistic Centre in New York prescribes chemotherapy in very low doses and raises the body temperature of his patients to 107.5°F by wrapping them in thermal blankets filled with water. And in Toronto a Dr Rudy Falk claims to have discovered a combination of heat and non-toxic drug which is remarkably successful. 'When I began,' he said, 'I thought it was a bunch of witchcraft' (*Toronto Saturday Star* May 29th 1982). It is interesting for one member of Cancer Contact to note that having been unable to sweat much most of her life, after secondary cancer was diagnosed she found that if she got so hot during the night wrapped in her duvet that she sweated profusely, she felt heaps better for it. Perhaps Dr Coley should be given a pardon, especially as we now know that out of 894 'hopeless cases' whom he treated, 426 had apparently survived and could still be traced between 5 and 80 years later (*Daily Express* November 23rd 1982).

Laws to prevent the public being led astray may have been necessary, and it was the Cancer Act of 1939 and the Medical Act of 1941 that made it illegal to advertise anything as a cure for cancer, TB or diabetes. There should perhaps also be a law to make it illegal to obstruct research into some of the alternative therapies both inside and outside the medical establishment.

Many alternative therapies are closely linked with the religious or philosophical beliefs of their originators, and this deters some sceptics from applying the scientific method when considering the claims made by the medically unorthodox. It is possible to be, as it were, superstitious upside down. If our established medical men and women are so scared, for instance, of walking under the ladder of Rudolf Steiner's discoveries that they can't even look up to see where they lead to, or look down to see if perhaps they are after all on firm ground, we shall miss Steiner's ecological good advice as well as his medical innovations. We may reject 99 per cent of Mary Baker Eddy's teaching in Christian Science without denying that she was right to stress the importance of mind over matter. You don't have to accept the Jewish faith in order to believe that 'Thou shalt love thy neighbour as thyself' (Lev. 19:18) and you don't have to be an atheist to agree with Bertrand Russell that 'What we need is not the will to believe, but the wish to find out'. When a number of intelligent, responsible, caring people 'find out' to their own satisfaction that some therapy or remedy reduces suffering — so long as they do not exploit their discovery financially or by making false claims — who dares openly to come down on the side of continued suffering? 'For the sick,' Hippocrates taught, 'the least is best', and today doctors still take the Hippocratic Oath: 'By Apollo, the physician, by Aesculapius, by Hygeae — by Panacea, and by all the gods and goddesses ... '

5. Mind Over Matter

Relaxation

Even if you are not tense before you are told you have cancer, you may well be so on hearing the news. Relaxation is perhaps the technique most of us need to learn first if we are to get the most out of other gentle therapies. There are many different methods described in books or on cassettes, but it is a great help to practise it with others, with an expert leading you through the process. Some members of Cancer Contact studied 'Mental Ataraxis', taught by Dr Ainslie Meares to the group's 'great sustainer', Lee. Dr Meares practised as a psychiatrist for 30 years and retired from medicine in order to study the effect of intensive meditation on cancer growth. His book *The Wealth Within* is an excellent introduction, and in it he reminds us that although it is unreasonable to expect dramatic changes at the first attempt, Mental Ataraxis is 'not a tedious business requiring months of practice'.

Deep relaxation and meditation are closely linked, the aim being to still the thinking mind and shift the awareness from the rational to the intuitive mode of consciousness. Some people achieve this by concentrating on their breathing; some repeat a word they find helpful (there is nothing 'magic' about a mantra!); others may concentrate on a visual symbol like a burning candle or a mobile. Anything in fact that helps relaxation, which is usually easier to achieve physically than mentally. Bio-feedback gadgets can be a great help by registering the level of relaxation reached, and reminding you to focus on specific points of tension such as the jaw, neck and shoulders.

The rhythmical movements of T'ai Chi Chuan and Hindu Yoga can lead to the same feeling of peace and serenity.

There is no harm in making the process easier by treating stress and tension homoeopathically, and with Dr Bach remedies.

Visualisation or Imagery Therapy

There was a jingle in the 1930s which went something like this: 'Every day in every way I'm getting better and better', although I can't remember if health or morals were implied. Visualisation therapy today is a form of auto-suggestion or self-hypnosis; an exercise in positive thinking on the assumption that if you start driving convinced that you will fail your test, you probably will fail it. Similarly, if you imagine vividly enough your immune system defeating your cancer, it may help to do so.

Dr Carl Simonton, co-founder and director of the Cancer Counselling and Research Center in Dallas, Texas, has introduced thousands of practitioners in many countries to his method of using relaxation and visualisation for self-healing. Since 1971 he and his daughter Stephanie have had some failures but also many successes: one of the first was with a man who had been suffering from impotence for 20 years; he also had arthritis. Both were cured. The Simontons believe that if nothing else they can improve the quality of their patients' experiences: for some their survival span has been doubled. Although people are encouraged to take responsibility for their own health, there are no attempts to induce feelings of guilt.

To practise the visualisation therapy you need to be relaxed, so that the imagination can concentrate all its energy — first on visualising the cancer in your body at its nastiest, and then going on to imagine the cancer cells being attacked by almost anything you like. The attackers could be lively white blood corpuscles pouring in to overcome the enemy, an avalanche of snow, white ballet skirts whirling round, people in white overalls with brooms, or white sharks hungry to gobble up the disease; leaving the body clean and healthy. Or it might be a white searchlight; everything flooding, moving, spinning in such a way as to drive the cancer out of the body. From there you go on to imagine yourself at your healthiest, happiest and most active. If you find it hard to move around, think of yourself walking with ease. If you are in pain, imagine it as a fiery ball and a great white sponge coming in to mop it up and take it away. Imagine yourself without pain, scars or disability. It is not always easy. One member of Cancer Contact found that when she was depressed she could not imagine anything white at all; everything was black. So change the imagery; imagine the blackness being rolled up in a sheet of some lighter colour, or drench it with a sparkling shower of rain turning to sleet or snow. People who have lost their pituitary glands may find it impossible to imagine anything at all, but with the gland, practice and luck, visualisation therapy can help to rid you of negative thoughts and resentments. *Getting Well Again* by C. Carl Simonton, Stephanie Matthews-Simonton and James L. Creighton is an excellent introduction to this therapy. It was an orthodox GP who gave it to a member of Cancer Contact, where it soon became the group's 'bible'.

Hypnotherapy

The media have given hypnosis by practitioners a bad name, but healing by therapists through the use of the hypnotic condition can be useful for those suffering from anxiety, emotional problems in general, or difficulty with giving up smoking. The patient stays wide awake and is put into a peaceful relaxed state; the words of the hypnotherapist are aimed at changing attitudes and states of mind that cause phobias and other problems.

The principal association of private psychotherapists in Great Britain is the National Council of Psychotherapists, which was formed in 1970. All members subscribe to a code of ethics similar to that of any branch of the medical profession. The therapist is forbidden to enter into contracts with patients, to accept gifts or to allow personal relationships to develop. The therapist also undertakes to terminate treatment at the earliest possible moment. Complaints are dealt with promptly and, if it is necessary, are referred to a disciplinary committee.

Further information from:
National Council of Psychotherapists, 1 Clovelly Road, Ealing, London W5 (tel. 567 0262); Gilbert Anderson LCNP, The Anderson-Hart Cancer Research Project, 2 Overbury, Middlesex Road, Bexhill-on-Sea, East Sussex TN40 1LP; Dr Alec Forbes, Cancer Help Centre, Grove House, Cornwallis Grove, Clifton, Bristol BS8 4PG (tel. Bristol 743216); John Beard FNCP, The Glebe House, Church Lane, Pevensey, East Sussex (tel. Eastbourne 762360 and 23055), who also has clinics in Brighton and Tunbridge Wells.

Healing

Dr Brian Josephson FRS, Regius Professor of Physics at Trinity College, Cambridge, 1973 Nobel prizewinner in physics who conducted a series of experiments with Matthew Manning in Toronto in 1974, wrote: 'I think we are on the verge of discoveries which may be extremely important for physics. We are dealing with a new kind of energy. This force must be subject to laws. I believe ordinary methods of scientific investigation will tell us a lot about psychic phenomena. They are mysterious, but they are no more mysterious than a lot of things in physics already.'

There appears to be enough evidence now to prove that some people, be they atheists or theists, have a natural ability to stimulate the body's own self-healing processes. The patient does not have to have 'faith'. When we remember that people use less than 20 per cent of their brain capacity, while neurologists have little idea what the unused parts of the brain are for, it is not surprising that even in scientifically controlled experiments physicists cannot understand or explain some of the things that other people make happen.

Healers like Matthew Manning, Gilbert Anderson and Paul Solomon have had many years of experience with cancer patients. Sometimes bio-feedback gadgets are used in conjunction with relaxation therapy. These are related to what we call 'lie detectors', by measuring skin resistance they can give an indication as to how deeply relaxed the patient is able to become.

Some healers claim to be able to take the cancer from the patient into themselves. In spite of the fact that they also insist that they can then banish the cancer altogether, it may be psychologically impossible for some people to believe in so many intangibles — from the power of the unexplained energy and that of the specific healer, to a certainty that you will not inflict your disease on them. Absurdities, however, do tend to vanish when survival is offered in the face of imminent death, and many people report having regained some degree of health without showing any signs of hysteria or emotional blackmail. One secular humanist is said to be able to practise healing, but with only one hand!

A Christian mother wrote a moving letter to the *Guardian* (June 29th 1983) describing how she and her husband had refused to arrange for the laying on of hands for their son, partly because the boy was an agnostic and was unconscious and could not be consulted. The parents felt that the prayers being offered for the boy's recovery should be enough. In spite of orthodox medical treatment and prayer the boy died, but the mother did not regret the decision they had taken. She wrote: 'What I do believe is, that if there is a God, He is not someone who can be bribed into granting special favours through prayer or by any other means, as pagans bribe their gods by sacrificing goats for better crops. If rituals such as the laying on of hands can help anyone come to terms with the illness or probable death of someone they love, then by all means let them continue to make use of them. But no one should suffer from the illusion that it will make any difference to the outcome. Some of those prayed for will recover: others will not. This is in accordance with natural laws; we should make greater efforts to improve medical knowledge, not rely on superstitious mumbo-jumbo. God surely would prefer us to act in this way.'

This letter draws attention to the difference between the 'laying on of hands' by clergymen who rely on the faith of the patient (and may have no natural ability to heal) and the work of people who claim no authority and may be surprised at what they find they are able to do. Given a rational and sceptical approach, the work of healers is worth exploring even if all else hasn't quite failed. But do check references.

World Federation of Healing, 134 Darnley Road, Gravesend, Kent DA11 0SN (tel. 0474-62304).

National Federation of Spiritual Healers, Old Manor Farm Studio, Church St, Sunbury-on Thames, Middlesex (tel. 09327-83164).

The New Age

Sooner or later students of alternative therapies (or 'holistic medicine' as they are sometimes called) may come across the 'New Age' philosophy, which goes back, we are told, to the all-male Jewish sect of the Essenes, and to the Egyptian Therapeutae. The New Age (according to those who believe in astrology) is the Age of Aquarius and the Second Coming, and some of its adherents believe that the Christ has already returned and is waiting to be discovered among the

Asians in London's East End. Jesus is seen as one of the 'Masters of Wisdom' — there are no 'Mistresses'.

The Essenes' working habit was white, and their descendants are referred to as 'the White Robed and Holy Ones from the Other Side'. Their white magic of prayer, fasting and baptisms was their 'therapy', but the cure was dependent on the sick person's degree of faith. The Essenes were also eclectics, however, and there is some religious and medical eclecticism in the New Age, but psychologically very little reference to Adler or Freud.

The 'White Brotherhood' included Rudolf Steiner, the White Eagle Lodge, the late Ronald Beasley, and a number of onco-therapists and doctors involved with the 'gentle method' of cancer treatment. Alice Bailey was also a leading figure, and her autobiography and other writings help to explain what the New Age is all about, with its middle-class apolitical conservatism and pre-Christian theosophy. Alice had an unloving father, a miserable childhood, a tormented adolescence, an unhappy marriage, divorce, and then relief only in her middle age from a vision of 'a tall well-dressed man in a turban' from Tibet, whose telepathic advice she spent the rest of her life passing on with an authority she had never previously achieved. To be a good occultist, she said, you had to be a practising mystic with 'the power to feel accurately', and she 'felt' she knew the Will of God like the back of her hand. At last this ugly duckling could claim to be 'superior in feeling and intuition' and no one could prove her wrong; they could only disagree with her and then she denounced them as 'silly idiots', and 'nincompoops' if they dared to claim that they too could communicate with the Masters. Nevertheless she continued to be haunted by fears, especially of death, and for this she found comfort in the hypothesis of reincarnation. Alice soon claimed to be one of her Master's senior disciples, and she opened her own school for pupils demanding entrance to 'the Mysteries' and wanting to learn to know God. 'Occult obedience' and 'physical purity' were part of the syllabus. Alice died (or, as her followers put it, 'gained her release from the limitations of the physical vehicle') in 1946.

New Age healing is achieved through what are called 'transmission groups', by using an instrument to which quartz crystals are attached by silver wires and laid on the patient's appropriate 'centres'. Each member of the group has to 'place the attention on the centre (chakra) between the eyebrows, without strain, and inwardly sound the mantra "OM", to hold it there'. Disease is stated to result from faulty attitudes of mind and wrong patterns of emotion, and to find out what are the 'right' patterns and attitudes you must, of course, ask the New Age and accept its authority. Discussion and argument is not encouraged, for 'when the right moment comes' everyone with any sense will see 'the Truth'.

The Aquarian Age has its own Gospel of Jesus the Christ, 'transcribed' by an American, Levi H. Dowling (1884–1911). Early in life he had been told in a vision to 'build a white city' and the gospel was it. In it we read: 'The fount of health is your soul: it has a door locked fast: the key is faith. And everyone can have this key and unlock the door and plunge into the healing fount and be made whole.' Levi adds: 'There is no deeper death than ignorance and unbelief.' So we are back with the Essenes and the idea that 'cure' depends on 'belief'. This is a dangerous maxim, of course, for it all depends on what we are asked to believe, and it is hardly fair to have to choose between being ill and forcing yourself to believe that something you find patently false, unethical or dishonest is true. It is with some relief that we turn to Gregory of Nazianzus who wrote to St Jerome in the 4th century AD: 'A little jargon is all that is necessary to impose on the people. The less they comprehend the more they admire. Our forefathers have often said, not what they thought, but what circumstances and necessity dictated.' Cancer patients know all about that!

Although the holistic healers have done notable work pioneering the complementary cancer treatments, and show an admirable ecological awareness, there is no doubt that their jargon can cause New Age tensions. Dr Steven Greer, a researcher in psychological medicine at King's College London, claimed to have found a clear link between breast cancer and 'extreme suppression of anger throughout adult life'. He believed he could predict the result of a biopsy accurately from psychological factors, and be correct 72 per cent of the time. What we also need to know of course is (a) what proportion of the population is able to avoid 'extreme suppression of anger' at home, at work, in sport, etc. and (b) how many people who suppress their anger to an extreme degree are nevertheless cancer-free.

Dr Greer's team also looked for biochemical explanation of their findings, and they concluded that anger-suppression produced a raised blood level of Immunoglobin A, which was also associated with cancers that spread to other parts of the body within a year of surgery to remove the original growth (i.e. the first growth to be diagnosed.) With this in mind we surely need research to find the effects of various cancer treatments and therapies (from radiotherapy and homoeopathy to Dr Bach) on Immunoglobin A.

The New Age oncologists can get quite angry themselves in their intolerance of philosophical materialism and secular humanism, but even in the cause of cancer prevention they do not seem to welcome the anger of those who feel that talk of 'karma' and 'the other side' is unlikely to contribute towards achieving co-existence between the orthodox and the unorthodox medical systems. It is not just being able to express one's own anger that is important, it is also the ability to welcome the anger of those who are angry with us.

Although individuals in Cancer Contact had studied the New Age, as a group we did not become involved but continued to concentrate on trying to achieve a lively, enjoyable and interesting Old Age for ourselves and for each other.

6. You Are What You Eat

The American doctor Richard Passwater was exposed to cancer-producing agents as a chemist working with insecticides and nerve gases, and was also receiving dangerous doses of radiation from X-ray equipment. He believes he has protected himself from cancer with diet and vitamins, and his book *Cancer and Its Nutritional Therapies* will, he hopes, help others to prevent as well as treat cancer. He writes: 'The goal is, of course, to combine the best of all therapies', but he adds that 'all are doomed without proper nutrition'. And so we are left with the question — 'what is proper nutrition for the cancer-conscious citizen?'

Walter de la Mare wrote: 'Whatever Miss T eats turns into Miss T.' If Miss T eats meals which cause obesity, overburden her liver, produce allergic symptoms, give her indigestion or make her feel or be sick, then her body cannot possibly be at the top of its healing form. Many of the oncologists in alternative medicine present their own pet theories as gospel truth, suggesting that if we ignore them then we deserve to be ill. There is no absolute truth about diets, however, not even for cancer. We have to make our way through all the confusing information and then decide to eat what makes us feel good; this means experimenting until we have discovered what it is we have eaten that made us feel bad. (Anyone intrigued by the links between 'good' and 'health', and 'bad' and 'disease', may find Samuel Butler's famous novel *Erehwon* amusing reading ...)

Most of the modern cancer diets have been influenced by Dr Max Gerson, the German physician who treated his first three cancer patients (all of whom had been diagnosed as 'terminal') in 1928. All recovered on his dietary treatment. Ten years later he was licenced to practise in New York and in 1946, he became the first physician to demonstrate recovered cancer patients before a US Congressional Committee. Gerson wrote: 'Cancer is an extraordinary symptom only. The underlying cause is to be found in the poisoning of the liver.' 'The more the whole body is detoxified, replenished and activated, the more the cancer is doomed' [24]. The Gerson therapy (we read) cannot usually succeed, however, if the patient is having 'chemotherapy, cortisone treatments, more than 16 cobalt or 40 X-ray treatments, etc., etc.' Even for those people who have avoided orthodox treatments the therapy is extremely demanding, especially on the meal-getters. For many people the cost and disciplines required alone make it impractical. But there is no doubt that it can work, as one friend of Cancer Contact proved by going to Mexico to the Gerson clinic. Her malignant melanoma has caused her no more trouble.

Carnivores versus Vegetarians: Without becoming a fanatic it is surely sensible to be aware of the drugs and hormones fed to cattle and poultry. Dr Dick Richards (author of *Topic of Cancer,* who has his own cancer clinic in Kent) recommends a Bio-Diet which, in the early stages, omits dairy produce and animal protein; but he is not a vegetarian himself and 'shoots for the pot', believing that wild meats like rabbit, pheasant and venison are good for health. He writes that people who think it wrong to kill for food may not hesitate to seize living plant matter and eat it when it's alive, and plants should be treated no worse than animals. There is at least a good discussion point there! In 1958 Max Gerson wrote: 'Without knowing it, many vegetarians today are "starving". The protein content of most vegetables and fruits went down in the last ten to twenty years, and we would have to make great efforts to bring it back to normal or even near normal.'

Mormons who eat a lot of meat have a lower cancer rate than Seventh-Day Adventists, who are usually vegetarians. Nevertheless many onco-nutritionists do recommend avoiding all meat, and it is said that when meat fat is heated to a very high degree methylcholanthrene can be formed, and this can cause cancer and also sensitise the body so that other carcinogens at a lower concentration cause cancer cells to form.

Even if meat were proved to be good for cancer patients, many people would still refuse to eat it for ethical reasons.

Dr E. Cuyler Hammond, one-time vice-president of the American Cancer Society, wrote: 'Much or perhaps most human cancer is caused not by single carcinogenic agents, but by interaction of multiple factors to which people are exposed.' ([46], p.41.) For instance nitrites (salt-like chemicals added to give meat colour and flavour and protect it and us from botulism) are not in themselves cancer-producing, but — when combined in the body with certain amines — nitrosamines are formed, and these are dangerous. The problem for food manufacturers is to use enough nitrites to prevent botulism without producing nitrosamines. Most onco-nutritionists advise us (especially when first diagnosed as having cancer) to avoid bacon, sausages, tinned and all dyed and processed foods. Vitamin C has been shown to block the formation of nitrosamines.

According to Dr James Thompson of Surrey

University, 'Only half of the 3,000 additives in use are useful; the others are only cosmetic to make something appear as it is not.' ([46], p.81.) Our governments have not been notable for banning pollutants, in agriculture, on the roads or elsewhere. One Canadian government official is quoted as saying: 'We don't know that much about cancer, how it is produced ... therefore, we can't be sure what is a safe level.' ([46], p.77.) Until we do, and while cancer continues in what are virtually epidemic proportions, we need to be on the safe side.

Recently in Puerto Rico little girls of four have begun to menstruate and a year-old baby developed her first ovarian cyst. As a result of the necessary surgery it is unlikely she will ever be able to have children of her own. Both little girls and boys have developed breasts. Dr Carmen Saenz (who documented 3,000 cases of this condition known as 'premature thellarche') has been fighting what is virtually a one-woman campaign for official action, believing that the cause lies in contaminated food, especially the illegal use of the female hormone oestrogen in poultry farming. The island also produces 90 per cent of birth control pills sold in the USA, and both male and female factory workers involved in their production suffer from swollen breasts and high cancer rates (*Channel 4 TV* June 1st 1983)

Dr Maud Tresillian Fere won her own battle against cancer of the bowel by following a strict salt-free diet. She is convinced that cancer is nearly always caused by excessive sodium in a person who has been debilitated by breaking the laws of health which she outlines in her book *Does Diet Cure Cancer?* What happens (she suggests) is this: an excess of salt (sodium) without any protective acid immediately joins with two-thirds of a molecule of water and forms caustic soda. *'This so irritates the body cells in that spot that they at once start to multiply'* (Fere's italics). At first the proliferation is slow and lactic acid in the body may neutralise the caustic soda, so that either a cancer tumour does not develop or a tumour grows but is benign. But trouble may begin as general health deteriorates. Alkalinity is a major problem in cancer patients (writes Dr Fere) and this can be tested by holding red litmus paper against the top gums for 3–4 minutes. This should stay red and not turn blue. Urine should also be slightly acid, but becomes alkaline after eating a lot of meat.

Horseradish is said to be effective for people who crave salt and find it very difficult to give up.

Dr Passwater warns against too many calories and too much polyunsaturated fat. He doesn't think cancer patients need worry much about cholesterol, saturated fats or, for that matter, meat. As he writes: 'A wise person learns to eat as many different foods as possible to allow the liver to detoxify each pollutant before it is stored in our fatty tissue. Eat well to keep your liver and immune system healthy. Eat as many unprocessed foods as you can. Wash your raw foods well. Avoid the foods that flagrantly pollute — especially dyed foods. Learn to read labels. Help your body work properly by maintaining a good activity (exercise) level' ([46], p.91).

Dr Dick Richards echoes the same commonsensical attitude. He answered the question 'Do patients revising their diet have to drink gallons of juices?' with 'Patients don't *have* to do anything. We have an armoury of weapons to fight the disease. We can use all or some ... the more we use, the more chance we have of winning the battle. Everything depends on what people can afford, availability and so on. I don't give orders' (*Here's Health,* June 1982).

The easiest way to avoid eating too many carbohydrates is to have a diet high in fat and high in proteins ([43], p.166). It's important to get enough protein at the beginning of the day. ([40], p.118). And the easiest way of eating an unhealthy diet is to be in hospital, which is really no place for anyone who is not 100 per cent fit. In 1979 a symposium ('Developments in Clinical Nutrition') at the Royal College of Physicians reported that 'many patients are starving in hospitals' and 'cancer patients, who particularly need balanced food regimes, are being treated like everyone else'. The working of the drugs might even be hindered by the malnutrition. Professor Johnstone of Newcastle University was reported as saying that hospital starvation 'can seriously damage a patient's chances of recovery ... doctors forget that the alimentary canal can collapse through lack of correct nutrition.' (*Sunday Times* June 10th 1979 and *Guardian* June 11th 1979).

Members of Cancer Contact had their own experiences of hospital diet with the regular supplies of carbohydrates, fibre-free meals, sausages, chips, ice cream and other sugary desserts. Even if this is 'what the doctor ordered', it is not what the patient should be having.

In 1983 it was revealed that a controversial report by a panel of leading doctors, scientists and food experts — commissioned by the government to recommend a healthier diet for the public — had been blocked for more than two years by the Department of Health. Much of the opposition to the report came from the British Nutrition Foundation which receives 98 per cent of its funds from the food manufacturing industry. The panel's findings have still not been published.

Most health food shops sell useful booklets on meatless recipes. Members of Cancer Contact found juices not only made them feel better, but tasted delicious: carrot and apple with bottled beetroot is one very useful one. They also sprouted their own seeds, so alfalfa and fenugreek and bean shoots could serve as salads especially during the winter months. Homemade yoghourt is much cheaper than that sold in the shops, and shop-bought yoghourt with added sugar bears little resemblance to the 'real thing'. Adelle Davis (and others) give recipes for specially nourishing 'potions' for faded appetites and weight loss.

The following is a very brief guide to a few useful books which can help to remove some of the alarm when considering changing eating habits and exploring the world of beans and pulses, sprouts and juices:

Susan E. Charmine: *The Complete Raw Juice Therapy* (Thorsons, 1981)

Adelle Davis: *Let's Get Well* (Unwin Books, 1974)

Rose Elliot: *The Bean Book* (Fontana, 1980)

Janet Hunt: *Simple and Speedy Wholefood Cooking* (Thorsons, 1982)

Cass McCallum: *Pulses, Seeds and Grains* (Molendinar Press, Glasgow, 1981). This book gives useful information as to what to do if you have forgotten to soak the beans.

Martha H. Oliver: *Add a Few Sprouts* (Pivot Books, USA, 1975)

Proteins are the main bearers of life. A full-grown human of about 60 kg needs some 60 grams of protein every day, and without sufficient ascorbic acid the cells cannot be put together correctly ([43], p.62). Half a cup of beans eaten with 1⅓ cups of rice gives the usable protein equivalent of a good-size steak. As cancers develop they take an ever-increasing amount of proteins from healthy tissue and (as Dr Passwater points out) *'Cancer patients usually die from wasting away, not from the size of the tumour.'* He quotes a Dr Stanley J. Udrick (University of Texas): 'Up until 1972 there was a taboo that if you fed a cancer patient you would accelerate the growth of the tumour. We've found this to be untrue.' Our immune systems, our defences and antibodies cannot function if deprived of proteins, calories, trace minerals and vitamins. So cancer patients should eat well — but wisely.

Carbohydrates should be strictly limited because cancer cells flourish on glucose. But it has to be remembered that starving the body in order to starve the cancer is not the answer.

Fats: A high fat diet is suspected of upsetting the hormone balance of the body and thereby contributing to cancer of the breast and prostate, and women who consume a lot of high fat dairy produce have a higher rate of breast cancer than women who eat a less rich diet (*Cancer Research* Sept. 1979; *Prevention* Vol 23/10).

There is of course a continuous battle between the butter producers and the manufacturers of margarine, and since 1976 there have been many medical reports to the effect that high cholesterol levels were killing off the human race by heart attacks. Vegetable oils and margarine high in polyunsaturated fats flooded the supermarkets and shopping baskets. It wasn't long, however, before these were themselves suspected of damaging the heart muscles and causing gall-stones and cancer of the bowel!

So what does the cancer patient do? As always: plough through the confusions, consider the vested interests of those giving advice, and choose as sensibly as possible. Drs W. Kaelin and R. Leroi, for instance, write in their *Special Diet:* 'Use butter or pure plant oils, such as cold pressed olive oil, sunflower seed oil, hazelnut butter. No margarine or mixed fats.'

There are two methods by which so-called 'cold pressed' oils are extracted from their parent seed. The oldest is the simple mechanical pressing (misleadingly called 'cold pressing' because no extra heat is applied). In fact the pressing itself produces some heat but the temperature is kept low so that vitamins are not destroyed. This method is used for soft, oily seeds such as olive, sunflower or sesame. The second method is the use of the screw or expeller press which is needed for harder seeds like safflower as well as for grains and beans from which the oil is difficult to extract. These 'unrefined oils' are rich in colour and fragrance and full of nutrients. They will keep for up to six months, and longer still if put in a sealed container in a dark place.

The so-called 'pure' and 'refined' oils, however, would go rancid immediately without the chemicals (usually petroleum based, such as benzine, hexane or heptane) which are added during processing. Oil companies say that the solvent residues are insignificant, but even small amounts of these substances can cause trouble: they can make blood cells deteriorate and speed up ageing. The process by which the 'crude' or 'unrefined' oil is 'refined' includes washing with caustic soda (which removes the valuable lecithin), bleaching, fine filtering (which destroys minerals) and deodorising by heating to a very high temperature. Refined oil is usually light in colour without any sediment or smell.

The following unrefined oils are recommended:
Corn germ oil — ideal for baking
Olive oil — for salads
Sesame oil — for everyday use
Sunflower oil — for sautéeing or deep frying
Safflower — (highest in polyunsaturated fats) for general use.

Bran is the outer part of the wheat which is removed during the milling of white flour; it helps absorb moisture in the gut. Surgeon Thomas Cleave RN fed his crew on the King George V battleship during the war on roughage and bran and was convinced that this is what kept them so fit. Mr Conrad Latto (consultant at the Royal Berkshire Hospital) stated some years ago that if everyone ate a small amount of bran every day, he and other surgeons specialising in bowel cancer (and diverticulosis) would soon be out of work.

It is interesting to note that one member of Cancer Contact was told to eat lots of white bread, white sugar, chicken, fish and sloppy foods for the few days before an operation in order to *inactivate* the bowel. He was forbidden to eat brown bread and bran, which promote normal bowel movements. Homemade bread with 100 per cent wholemeal flour, extra wheatgerm and sesame seeds makes a delicious basis for a healthy diet, and is much more satisfying than the equivalent amount of white Mother's Pride.

7. Vitamins and Other Substances

Patients should investigate vitamin dosage, and (whenever possible) find doctors who understand the importance of vitamin therapy in the treatment of cancer.

It has been estimated that some 65 million years ago our ancestors lost the ability to manufacture their own Vitamin C. Dr Newbold reckons that when we eat or crave for sweets today, we are really trying to get ascorbic acid. Some animals under stress can manufacture their own, from two to four grams a day, but this does not give them immunity to neoplasms (cancers). Human beings, guinea pigs and monkeys have to depend on a daily intake of Vitamin C, which is used up by the carcinogens that it helps to detoxify.

Albert Szent-Györgyi, the Hungarian who won the Nobel Prize in 1937 for isolating chemically pure Vitamin C, wrote: 'All living phenomena are to a great extent electronic phenomena. And cancer is also an electronic disease.' It is a defect in the 'electron transfer' in which Vitamin C is involved.

Linus Pauling says he doesn't believe that Vitamin C is a special anti-cancer wonder-drug, but that 'it works against cancer by bolstering the body's natural protective mechanisms in a number of different ways'. Allan Campbell, MD, FRCP, agrees that no one should be told that Vitamin C is a cure for cancer, but that 'ascorbic acid often greatly improves the quality of life of the cancer patient and helps him to live longer.' It is, then, a powerful back-up therapy and is not to be depised. Ewan Cameron (chief surgeon at the Vale of Leven Hospital, Lochlomondside, Scotland) has been treating cancer with Vitamin C since the early 1970s, and he believes that doctors should spend more time improving patients' resistance to cancer. If the body's level of Vitamin C is too low, the collagen will not be able to prevent the haphazard reproduction of the cells. Mr Cameron has measured the Vitamin C level in the serum and white blood corpuscles of many hundreds of cancer patients, and he has found that surgery, X-ray and cobalt treatment all lower the patients' levels of Vitamin C. He prescribes the fine-powder mixture of ascorbic acid, sodium ascorbate, or calcium ascorbate, depending on which type the patients can most easily tolerate. It is said that it is sometimes the 'binders' in Vitamin C tablets that can cause gastric trouble. It is worth trying to overcome such problems by one method or another, for as Albert Szent-Györgyi has written: Vitamin C is *'a substance which makes us sick by not eating it'*.

One of the first tests of people who appear to be resistant to cancer could surely be to see if they do in fact have high levels of ascorbic acid; the lack of it is believed by several members of Cancer Contact to have contributed to the appearance of their cancers. In 1976 it was reported that Vitamin C-treated breast cancer patients lived six times longer than their matched 'control' group, and Vitamin C-treated kidney patients lived five times longer' ([46], p.110), yet the National Cancer Institute continuously turned down Dr Pauling's request for research grants. In 1978 Pauling believed that Vitamin C could cut the cancer death rate by 75 per cent, but he was still unable to do proper research.If it is even remotely possible that Vitamin C acts as a de-toxifier, can (for instance) block the formation of nitrosamines in the body, can help relieve pain in the dying cancer patient, can kill cancer without affecting healthy cells by its own non-toxic chemotherapeutic action; if it makes patients feel better, and helps to protect them from infections, the disadvantages of surgery, radiotherapy and drugs, then what in the name of Marie Curie is preventing serious researchers from investigating, if it is not the pressures applied by the all-powerful drug companies?

And the dangers from Vitamin C? That the shrinking of the tumour might pull on a blood vessel and cause a haemorrhage; but presumably other attempts to shrink the tumours involve the same risk.

The Vitamin C disciples confirm Dr Fere's belief that cancer patients have little or no acid in their stomachs and that in order to get nutrition they have to have supplementary acids, preferably 60 minutes or so before a meal. And there is a bonus: high levels of ascorbate increase the body's tolerance of sodium. ([43], p.87.)

Allan Campbell writes how it is vitally important 'that the cancer patient be prepared for the onslaught of cancer treatment with proper nutrition, including large amounts of Vitamin C ... To jump in and give X-ray treatment and chemotherapy without paying special attention to the patients' nutritional needs is very bad' (ibid p.43). But that is exactly what happened to all the members of Cancer Contact. None was given any advice whatsoever about nutrition.

Vitamin C as a potential non-toxic anti-cancer agent is much too important to be ignored. Dr Linus Pauling sums up the situation for us when he says: 'I don't think that anything will ever replace surgery when the cancer is operable. However, I don't believe that there have been any thorough studies on Vitamin C as an alternative to high-energy radiation or the anti-cancer drugs. So, it will be necessary to make very careful studies of what the relationship of Vitamin C and other nutritional therapy is to these conventional treatments' ([46], p.112).

As for the dosage: this must be calculated for each individual, according to her or his need. The urine can be tested relatively easily to see how much Vitamin C is being excreted, but it must be remembered that this is no proof that the body is absorbing the vitamin adequately, and even on its way out it may well protect against cancer of the bowel and bladder. Six grams of Vitamin C a day is not seen as excessive by the Marsden Hospital. Some doctors recommend very much more.

Vitamin A was discovered in 1913 and can exist in several related forms. It is stored in the liver as 'retinol' and a link has been found between the retinol levels in the blood and the incidence of cancer.

When in June 1982 the National Academy of Sciences (USA) issued some guidelines for reducing cancer risks through diet, it concentrated on (a) a reduction in the intake of all fats, whether saturated or polyunsatured; (b) a reduction in the intake of alcohol, and (c) an increased intake of fruits, wholegrain cereal products and vegetables, especially those high in carotene which converts to Vitamin A. Beta carotene is one of the pigments which makes apricots, oranges and carrots the colour they are. If too much Vitamin A is taken, the liver may be damaged and the excess free retinol spill into the blood with potentially fatal consequences.

So what is 'too much'? When it comes to supplements, it depends of course on how much Vitamin A you are also taking in your diet, but Earl Mindell [40] says: 'More than 100,000 IU daily can produce toxic effects in adults if taken for many months' (and for infants more than 18,500 IU daily can be dangerous). Cancer patients should, as always, ask for advice from a qualified onco-nutritionist. Vitamin A deficiency may not in itself cause cancer, but it makes the mucous membranes less able to resist the disease, and stress depletes our supply of the vitamin.

As megadoses of vitamins may affect laboratory tests, it is always best to tell your doctors how many pills (and what sort) you have been taking, although many doctors sadly imagine that if cancer patients eat what is loosely called 'a good diet' they do not have to take any special care with their meals. A 'good diet', however, is nothing like as easy to provide these days as it used to be, before there was intensive food production and consumer seduction by the manufacturers.

Doctors who specialise in nutrition are not always experts when it comes to the best diet for you as a cancer patient. The Bristol Cancer Help Centre has produced some booklets with useful information about which vitamins to avoid. Women with breast cancer for instance are warned *not* to take Vitamin E, because of its hormone-like action, and there are also restrictions put on Vitamins B 6, B 12 and folic acid, which are said to enhance growths.

In spite of the evidence to show that aluminium (from cooking utensils, kettles, teapots and so on) and also many drugs hinder the absorption of vitamins, and that X-rays break down the body's proteins, producing histamine with resultant allergic effects, some doctors remain uninterested in the dangers cancer patients are running when it comes to destroying what at least *ought* to be good in their diets. Such a lack of interest from the medical profession is hard to understand. In his *Overfed but Undernourished* H. Curtis Wood wrote: 'Because of the remarkable advances that have been made in chemistry, it is now possible to synthesize many of the vitamins and mineral compounds that are used as food supplements. There is a difference of opinion as to whether the artificial product is as well utilised in the human body as is the natural or organic one. The problem is quite similar to that of organic farming or gardening — the ideal method is not always possible from a practical standpoint' ([57] p.83). Theron G.

Randolph however, the eminent allergist, wrote in *Chemical Environment:* 'A synthetically derived substance may cause a reaction in a chemically susceptible person when the same material of natural origin is tolerated, despite the two substances having identical chemical structures.' There seems evidence, then, to indicate that the biological activity of synthetic and natural vitamins is not identical. If we can get the natural vitamins on prescription, so much the better. The cost of being an intelligent cancer patient bent on survival can be very heavy. Good health should surely not in this day and age be a privilege only of those who can afford it. This is not what the pioneers of public medicine and national health services intended.

Minerals

Homoeopaths have been using selenium, gallium, arsenic and platinum in their treatment of cancer for more than a hundred years. When our immune system fails to protect us it may either be because we are deficient in this or that nutrient or because, although we have enough of them, our bodies are unable to absorb and make good use of these nutrients. The fact that such a minute homoeopathic dose of minerals has such a powerful effect may be partly because it stimulates the body's own supply, activating our own defences to protect us and defeat disease.

Dr Passmore believes that selenium deficiency is especially noticeable in women with breast cancer, but this mineral in allopathic doses can be toxic. In July 1983 it was reported in the *Lancet* that an American survey has shown that selenium is important in the prevention of cancer for men as well as for women. Indeed, the analysis suggests that those on a selenium-deficient diet may be six times more likely to develop cancer than those with an adequate selenium diet' (*Guardian* July 18th 1983). Other scientists doubt this, and the Harvard School of Public Health suggest that 'above a relatively low level, the presence of additional selenium has no protective effect'. Homoeopathic doses, then, may well be enough.

Iodine is also said to be deficient in many women with breast cancer, and without iodine oestrogen (which tends to be carcinogenic or at least co-carcinogenic) stays in the body longer. Iodine is also prescribed by homoeopaths for breast cancer.

Zinc is very important to the immune system, which is impaired by a low level of it. Dr Hans Nieper writes: 'The more lymphocytes which act against cancer cells, the more safety we have against cancer growth. Zinc orotate greatly activates the development of T-lymphocytes and increases their number, especially when a large amount of Vitamin A is given at the same time. Both Vitamin A and zinc are essential ingredients the thymus gland needs to inform lymphocytes to fight cancer cells' ([46], p.187). Again homoeopathic zincum metallicum is an effective drug for those whose symptoms fit.

Iron is a different kettle of metal. Iron supplements are often considered very dangerous for cancer patients, and this was reported in the *Lancet* in the late 1970s.

According to Leon Chaitow, most minerals should be taken as orotates or in a chelated form. His book *An End To Cancer?* contains much useful material.

It is difficult for patients to find out which (if any) vitamin or mineral deficiencies they are suffering from. There are however blood, sweat and hair tests carried out by the London Clinic at the request of a doctor: these are swiftly done but cost £40. For a hair test only the charge is £15. Hair tests are also organised by Biomed International at East Grinstead in Sussex; these are sent to Canada and inevitably take more time, costing over £20.

Enquiries at a local hospital from Cancer Contact

drew a patronising blank. Even if doctors agreed to request such tests, they are expensive and the NHS is short of money. Sometimes the response was in fact derision. It was not encouraging.

There are, however, doctors specifically involved with such tests: Dr Alan Stewart, M.F. Hom., at the Clinic of Natural Medicine in Hove, Sussex, and Dr Andrew Lockie, M.F. Hom., of Ealing and Guildford are firm believers in hair tests, for although blood samples show what is in the body at the time, and urine what is being expelled from it, two inches of hair provide an accurate record of what has been stored in the body for the previous four months. People who have had their hair bleached or 'permed' have to wait several months before asking to be tested.

As happens so often, it appears to be a lack of concern, interest and information that prevents the NHS providing preventive measures. The message is — wait until you have got cancer, and then we can write you off and get on with our really important work!

Enzymes

In order for our food to be satisfactorily digested it has to be chemically simplified. Enzymatic action breaks down the nutrients into smaller and simpler chemical fragments so that they can be absorbed through the walls of the 30-foot long digestive tract and thus enter the bloodstream. The enzyme 'ptyalin' in the saliva, for instance, splits starches into simple sugars, 'lipase' breaks down fats, and 'pepsin' in the stomach deals with meats and other proteins. The stomach of course is not indispensable to digestion, most of which occurs beyond it. Enzymes, then, are important catalysts. They are best obtained from uncooked and unprocessed fruits, vegetables, eggs, meat and fish, but are destroyed under certain heat conditions. As Earl Mindell [40] writes, one enzyme cannot substitute for another: 'A deficiency, shortage or absence of one single enzyme can mean the difference between sickness and health.' He warns that the label 'enriched' on foods can be very misleading and justifies the use of supplements in his very clear account of the digestive processes which are of vital importance to cancer patients.

Laetrile

Amygdalin or Laetrile (LAEvomandelonTRILE-beta-glucoside or Mandelonitrile glucoronide) has been the subject of much discussion. Dr Ernest T Krebs Snr has been working in the USA with this substance since 1923, and with his sons he perfected Laetrile in 1952. Krebs believes that cancer is caused by malfunctions of normal mechanisms within the body itself, and that these are the result of a deficiency in a chemical substance found in some foods, and of a deficiency in certain enzymes produced in the pancreas. The natural chemical food factor is 'nitriloside', and the enzymes are 'trypsins'. Krebs calls this chemical 'Vitamin B 17'; others say that this is not an accurate label.

Nitriloside contains cyanide, which is released only in the presence of an enzyme group called beta glucosidase or glucoronidase. This enzyme group is found to an appreciable extent only in cancer tissue. When it is found elsewhere, it is always accompanied by larger quantities of 'rhodanese', another enzyme, which is able immediately to render the cyanide harmless. Cancer tissue contains no rhodanese. Dr John A Richardson — incidentally, a member of the infamous John Birch Society — has been at the forefront in the Laetrile controversy in the USA, and writes: 'Cancer cells are faced with a double threat: the presence of one enzyme causes them to be exposed to cyanide, while the absence of another enzyme (which is found in all other cells) results in a failure to detoxify'

([49] p.4). The purpose of Laetrile, then, is to destroy cancer cells which, because of their composition, cannot withstand the cyanide, leaving the non-cancer cells unharmed.

This part of the body's defence system against cancer cannot work without a diet containing an adequate supply (whatever that is) of Laetrile, and if the pancreas is weak or exhausted by too much sugar or animal protein (says the doctor) the enzyme cannot do its job properly.

Laetrile is found in sesame seeds, alfalfa, chick peas, lentils, apricot, plum, peach stones and pear seeds as well as in many wild berries and brown rice among many other foods. It is being used in 28 or more countries as a treatment for cancer, and the alternative oncologists who have studied it appear convinced of its value, *so long as it is given under medical supervision.* Nevertheless there has been a bitter and ugly campaign against the treatment. Dr Richardson quotes a woman who went for her Laetrile injection and afterwards found the windscreen of her car engraved with 'You are going to die!' The campaign against this doctor began in 1971 after he had been in practice for 20 years as a GP and ENT specialist. He had treated many cancers with orthodox methods which (he writes) 'seldom prolonged the lives of my patients and in fact often seemed to shorten them. They hardly seemed worth the cost to the patient either in terms of financial outlay or in suffering from the painful side-effects of radiation burns and toxicity'. Having met Dr Krebs and studied the subject, Richardson became convinced by the theoretical evidence. What he needed was practical experience. In the USA there is a so-called 'Anti-Quackery Law'. Richardson says he 'never dreamed how much latitude was allowed to administrative public servants to define what was and what was not worthless; and never in my wildest imagination did I suspect that a multi-billion dollar drug industry had such influence over regulatory agencies of government as to constitute a virtual blockade against the development of drugless medicine'. Gradually he came to accept that cancer was not just a tumour, but a 'systemic condition'; by attacking only symptoms he and others in the medical profession had been ignoring the disease (or as Hahnemann would have said the 'sick people').

Dr Richard Passwater says that the American public knows that it has been lied to by those who have condemned Laetrile. In Britain, Dr Alec Forbes of the Bristol Cancer Help Centre claims that the trials were designed to fail, and the fact was that Amygdalin did help defeat cancer (*Guardian* February 9th 1983).

Amygdalin has been listed for over a hundred years in the United States Pharmacopeia as a non-toxic substance, yet one reason given for refusing to grant permits to carry out tests is that Laetrile might be toxic. In October 1983 it was reported that two people were unconscious for four hours after eating 20 apricot kernels each. This was 'very close to a lethal dose', said Mr Bob Edlin, deputy chief environmental health officer for Welwyn and Hatfield District Council (*Guardian* October 18th 1983). But as Dr Richardson writes: 'To deny permission to test on the grounds that amygdalin *may* be toxic is mind-boggling when one realises that virtually all drugs currently approved by the FDA (Federal Drug Administration) for cancer therapy are *extremely toxic.*'

We have had surgery since the year dot, radiation since the 1800s and chemotherapy since 1943, but still the cancer death rate goes up each year. As Richardson states: 'Orthodox medicine does *not* have the answer.'

People who want to try Amygdalin/Laetrile should contact a doctor who understands it and will prescribe; for instance:

The Cancer Help Centre, Grove House, Cornwallis Grove, Clifton, Bristol BS8 4PG (tel. Bristol 743216).

Dr Dick Richards, Kent Private Clinic (supervision

only), Sandwich, Kent CT13 9DL (tel. 0304-612910).

Herbalism

Herbalists use non-poisonous herbs in order to eliminate toxins from the body and also to nourish and revitalise it. It should not be forgotten, however, that herbs taken indiscriminately in large (allopathic) doses or for long periods can be toxic. If taken together with orthodox drugs the result might be an 'overdose', or the benefit of one or the other may be lost. Liquorice, for instance, may raise the blood pressure, so is best avoided by anyone with hypertension. Expert advice is needed. Members of the National Institute of Medical Herbalists (MNIMH) take a four-year training and, like many other unorthodox practitioners, treat the person rather than the disease.

Cancer patients may be advised to use fruit and vegetable juices and herbal teas as a daily means of detoxifying themselves, and these can be very effective. Those who take beetroot juice should not forget the fact when noticing what at first seems to be blood in the stools or urine. Jason Winters [60] was a 'terminal' cancer patient given three months to live. He survived, he claims, thanks to a herbal tea for which he found the recipe himself. There is no denying it tastes rather as one imagines tea made from mattress filling might taste, but it helps some people and makes them feel better. Red clover tea is also prescribed by herbalists; it was suggested to one of the Cancer Contact group that she should find a field, grow and cultivate her own, which cheered her up a lot as she didn't think she was going to live long enough to harvest the crop! Jason Winters', clover, camomile, fennel, lime ... any tea which lacks tannin is worth trying.

H.H. Zeylstra, MNIMH, 148 Forest Road, Tunbridge Wells, Kent (send a large s.a.e. for register of qualified practitioners).

Evening Primrose Oil

Dr Richaard Passwater comments [47] that although the idea of destroying pre-cancerous cells before they form a fully-fledged cancer is not a new approach, reversing cancer cells back to normal cells is. The rational way to do this is by techniques which cannot harm normal tissues. Dr David Horobin wrote in *Medical Hypothesis* that 'we already have the necessary information for this to be carried out'. Cancer cells are already defective, and it is when their proliferation rate exceeds their death rate that cancers grow. If proliferation can be controlled by normalising cell function, then the cancer cells will die and the cancer regress.

One use of Evening Primrose Oil may be to enhance the action of Vitamin C. Trials on this are taking place in the USA. Women who suffer from mastitis, however, may find that Evening Primrose Oil helps to prevent the development of cysts and remove existing lumps. This was discovered by accident when the oil was given to large numbers of women for other reasons. The disappearance or softening of the cysts occurred within a two to four month period. This may or may not be of direct interest to cancer patients, but any means of preventing the pain of mastitis and the fear that the existence of any breast lumps brings, is worth considering.

Urine Therapy

This had been publicised in the magazine *Woman,* and aroused some interest. Advocates suggest that the valuable minerals and salts in the urine can cure all manner of things, and the taking of it is quite harmless. Urine is sterile when it leaves the body but quickly decomposes, so it should be drunk immediately, if drunk at all. Cancer Contact members decided that even with orange juice they would rather wait a while.

The chief exponent in Britain is a Canadian-born osteopath, Arthur Lincoln Pauls, but another osteopath, the late Leslie O. Korth from Tunbridge Wells, told an interesting story of a woman with advanced breast cancer for whom a urine poultice applied three times a day had worked wonders. Applied externally to wounds and burns or sunburn, urine is said efficiently to remove pain and irritation. Sarah Miles published her own account of success with urine injections (very expensive in Los Angeles). She takes her own at home — in apple juice ...

8. Using Your Body

The Alexander Principle

Frederick Matthias Alexander (1869-1966) believed that good health is a matter of psycho-physical co-ordination which we have as young children and lose as we grow up, but which we can re-learn through educated sensory perception. It is not strictly a 'therapy', but a method of undoing ('inhibiting' as he put it) bad postural habit. There are no exercises to learn, only a new habit of *thinking* the body into a way of moving, sitting, lying, working, so that the maximum effect is gained with the minimum amount of energy. Just by saying 'I'm not going to clench my jaw, tighten my neck or hold my breath', we automatically help the body to function at its best, and with proper muscular adjustment the mind is at its most alert. Poise and a sense of general well-being is the hallmark of the proficient Alexander exponent, and it is claimed that many diseases can be prevented by those who master the technique. The *British Medical Journal* concluded: 'Alexander's work is of first-class importance, and investigation by the medical profession is imperative.'

The Nobel prizewinner Nicholas Tinbergen devoted his Nobel oration in 1973 to the subject.

Dr Wilfred Barlow wrote [1]: Any investigation into problems of "dis-ease" and "de-vitalisation" must take into account the persistent influence of USE in every reaction and during every moment of life. Any diagnosis which ignores this influence is incomplete. Any plan of treatment with fails to take it into account must leave behind a predisposition to disease and malfunctioning' (p.94). 'There are no diseases,' (he adds) 'only sick people.' And sick people suffering from hypertension (high blood pressure) and all the other ailments in which stress is an obvious factor can benefit from learning the Alexander technique which, however (like all other worthwhile and long-lasting skills), demands application and a lot of practice. It is the way we 'use' our bodies every minute of the day that determines whether or not we stay healthy. Cancer patients have at least seen the red light.

Details from: The Secretary, Alexander Institute, 36 Albert Court, Prince Consort Road, London SW7.

Osteopathy

The practice of osteopathy goes back to America in the 1870s, when A.T. Still (who had attended a short course at the Kansas College of Physicians and Surgeons) insisted that he had set 17 dislocated hips in 24 hours. He started an osteopathic medical college which by 1902 had 500 students. 'Dr' Still was soon condemned as a quack, partly because he claimed 100 per cent cures. One of his patients, a Daniel Palmer, started a clinic of his own and his form of manipulation became known as Chiropractic. Many doctors treat osteopaths as if they are no more qualified than Still, but today they undergo four years of training and, apart from surgery and drugs, they are as medically trained as doctors and are qualified to diagnose. They would lose this right, however, if they worked within the NHS. They can receive patients directly, without reference from a medical practitioner, although many doctors will now recommend osteopathy which covers treatment of disturbance of function, not only in the spine but in organs of the body.

Osteopaths use their own kinds of manipulation for many ailments, and by no means only dislocated joints. For instance they can stimulate the movement of lymph through the lymph nodes and so help the healthy production of antibodies, which may prove healing for infectious diseases. One American osteopath, Marvin H. Soalt of New Jersey, takes blood and hair analysis and works out diets for his patients on a computer.

It was William Garner Sutherland (1873-1954), an American osteopath, who observed that the living skull is not a rigid, solid unit, but that the bones fit together, each of them surrounded by a layer of membrane which allows a very slight amount of movement between them. This flexibility had been overlooked by the medical profession, and Sutherland had himself been taught that no movement was possible in the sutures of the cranium. As he began to question the reasons for the design of the skull, he found that no one was interested and he received no help in the research he was determined to carry out.

Continuing with his observations alone, Sutherland discovered that good physical and mental health depends not only on the position of the cranial bones, but also on their freedom of movement. He began to teach his theories in the 1940s, and his students were able to see for themselves that restrictions (due to injury or disease) of the normal movement caused many health problems. He formulated a concept based on his important physiological discoveries. These include:

1) The inherent mobility of the brain and spinal cord.
2) The fluctuation (tidal flow or movement) of the cerebrospinal fluid.
3) The mobility of the reciprocal tension membrane

(Dura Mater) within the skull and spine.
4) The articular mobility of the cranial bone.
5) The involuntary mobility of the sacrum (triangular bone above the coccyx).
For a person to be healthy, all these units must function harmoniously.

Without X-rays or other tests cranial osteopaths can often, by the trained sensitivity of the fingers and hands, diagnose and treat the malfunctioning of some organ or tissue deep within the body, and they have an uncanny way of detecting a patient's problem whether it be depression or some long past injuries. Because the treatment involves a minimal amount of very gentle physical adjustment (this is so slight that the patient is hardly aware of anything at all being done), this can be especially valuable for people in pain, the root of which often lies in the connective body tissue (the fascia), the links between the bones, muscles and so on. Any abnormal tightening (including shrinking by radiotherapy) exerts a pull on another part of the body structure. This is why an injury to the lower back can cause headaches, or radiotherapy cause muscular pain. Craniosacral treatment can provide much relief.

Osteopaths study cranial osteopathy as post-graduates, but not all who take this training go on to practise it. The best way to find a practitioner is to contact the General Council and Register of Osteopaths, 1-4 Suffolk Street, London SW1Y 4HG (tel: 01-839-2060) or phone a local registered osteopath for advice. Your local library should have a copy of the register of osteopaths qualified to give treatment; beware those who are not qualified. Some people learn manipulation, but are quite unqualified to know when (and — just as important — when not) to use it.

Acupuncture

Acupuncture is a method of healing which has been used in China for more than 3,000 years. It is claimed that it works by manipulating the 'Chi' or life energy which is the vital force in all living things, and flows around the body in what are called 'meridians'; if these get blocked because of some constitutional problem, stress or even weather, there is an imbalance of energy which needs correcting if the body's healing processes are not to be hindered. With the appropriate stimulation the white blood cells can be released so as to fight off disease, calcium deposits can be dealt with, and circulation improved. Once banished by acupuncture, it is claimed, the disease should not appear again.

The acupuncturist will go into all the details of a patient's situation: most important, s/he will take the pulses on each wrist (six on each side) and from this a diagnosis will be made. The state of the 'Chi' in the 12 meridians will be known.

Treatment consists of inserting some small needles, quite often (but not always) painlessly. These are left in for about 20 minutes. During the course of treatment, diseases may reappear which had been absent for 20 years or so; this is because one disease evolves into another, and in order to achieve a full cure, they all have to be removed like taking off the layers of an onion. Some people, however, do not respond to treatment. Like homoeopathy, acupuncture can work with animals as well as humans, which proves that it is not faith healing. Generally three to six weekly visits are necessary, and as the patient improves, the treatments are gradually spread out.

The proof that it works? There have been thousands of experiments, but one which seems irrefutable has shown that acupuncture can cause a significant increase in the white cell count. This is, of course, of interest to cancer patients as to everyone else. It is illegal to claim that anything at all can 'cure cancer', but acupuncturists certainly claim to be able to cure nearly everything else! It is worth investigating.

Acupressure Techniques: These are usually defined as being 'for the self-treatment of minor ailments' but are no less interesting to those with major problems. Dr Hans Ewald [21], for instance, gives simple diagrams of where to apply finger pressure (and for how long) in order to relieve fatigue, various forms of pain, anxiety and even tobacco addiction. A member of Cancer Contact was able to hold at bay an attack of migraine in a friend who had to drive home: she was able to drive and the vomiting was delayed until she was in the right place. The system is so simple that anyone can follow it and if it doesn't work there is still no harm done. If it does — another extremely grateful person.

The British Acupuncture Association, 34 Alderney Street, London SW1 will provide lists of practitioners; finding out about how qualified or reputable they are is not so easy. Unfortunately, there are many people who call themselves 'doctor' when they have no medical training.

T'ai Chi Chuan (also spelt Taijiquan)

In China and Chinese communities elsewhere people of all ages can be seen, often early in the morning and outdoors, going through a series of slow, flowing and graceful movements known as T'ai Chi. This is a system of moving meditation. Master T.T. Liang writes [35]: 'Of all the exercises, I should say that T'ai Chi is the best. It can ward off disease, banish worry and tension, bring improved physical health and prolong life. It is a good hobby for your whole life; the older you are, the better. It is suitable for everyone — the weak, the sick, the aged, children, the disabled and blind.' All you need is a space three feet square. Everything is done very slowly and gently: the aim — mental and physical balance. Like the Alexander principle, T'ai Chi puts great emphasis on moving in ways which allow the maximum of effect for the minimum amount of energy. As with yoga and other meditative systems it is necessary to learn the appropriate breathing, and this can prove especially helpful to those who find relaxation difficult.

Traditionally T'ai Chi has been linked with the Taoist philosophy and also with the traditional Chinese understanding of medicine, with its emphasis on the flow of healing energy (the 'Chi') in mind and body. Although the People's Republic of China today doesn't entirely approve of the philosophical or medical ideas, T'ai Chi (like acupuncture) continues to be encouraged because of its proven benefits to health.

The student of T'ai Chi is usually taught a 'form' which consists of a sequence of movements which flow into one another and last about ten minutes. Once this has been learnt, it becomes the basis of practice and improvement. Better breathing, suppleness, physical relaxation and a meditative state of mind are the rewards.

It is best to learn T'ai Chi from an experienced teacher. Contact the British T'ai Chi Chuan Association: 7 Upper Wimpole Street, London W1M 7TD (tel: 01-935-8444).

Yoga

'Yoga' means 'to yoke', or as E.M. Forster put it, 'only connect'. It is at least 4,000 years old and possibly a thousand years older than that. Basically it is a system of bodily and mental discipline which aims to achieve self-realisation or spiritual illumination. There are many different kinds of yoga and many different kinds of teachers. Vivekananda, for instance, warned against 'life negation'. Meditation, he said, should not lead to introspective egoism. 'Here is the world, and it is full of misery. Go out into it as Buddha did, and struggle to lessen it or die in the attempt. Forget yourselves: this is the first lesson to be learnt, whether you are a theist or an atheist, whether you are an agnostic or a Vedantist, a

Christian or a Mohammedan' (*Practical Vedanta*). [27]

Raja Yoga aimed to 'check the flow of thought' and to still the mind from concentration, on the principle that when the mind is relaxed and held steady it is at its most receptive and creative, and problems are most easily solved. Hewitt claims [27] that 'Yoga is the most practical available means of attaining health and happiness in an age of stress.'

Cancer patients, however, especially if they have other problems like high blood pressure or arthritis, should be very careful to make sure that what they try to do will not do more harm than good. It is essential to begin yoga postures with relaxation and breathing. Osteopaths see many patients who come to them because they have tried to do yoga while cold, stiff and brittle.

Reflexology

This is a method of foot massage which sounds absurd — until it is tried. A sceptical nurse who had been constipated for ten days had to run for the lavatory because of its effect. Pain, which nothing else (including orthodox drugs) is able to shift, can be relieved by a skilful and (of course) trained therapist. We can also do it for ourselves (so long as we can reach our feet and have the strength in our hands to apply quite firm pressure in the tender areas). There are excellent books describing the technique, and there are reflexologists in many areas of the country.

International Institute of Reflexology,
PO Box 34, Harlow, Essex.
The Bayly School of Reflexology,
Monk's Orchard, Whitbourne, Worcs.

9. Pain and Hospices

People unable to experience pain are in great danger: in leprosy they can lose fingers without knowing it. Mary Baker Eddy (founder of Christian Science) said that because we are created in the image of the Divine Mind (which knows no pain), pain does not exist. In reply 'Anon' wrote:

> There was a faith-healer of Deal
> Who said 'Although pain isn't real,
> If I sit on a pin
> And it punctures my skin
> I dislike what I fancy I feel.'

Most of us accept pain as a useful but unpleasant reality, and the orthodox method of dealing with it is by drugs, which all too often cause a miserable mental confusion and muddled memory. There are alternative methods which may be as successful and avoid the side-effects, as have already been described — homoeopathic remedies, acupuncture and acupressure, reflexology, cranial osteopathy, hypnosis and visualisation therapy.

The body, however, also has its own protection — the 'endorphines' which set out to block the pain messages being relayed to the rest of the body, and these natural pain-killers may be stimulated by the alternative therapies. There is also an opiate antagonist — 'naloxene' — which in its turn blocks the production of endorphines. Maybe it is an excess of naloxene which causes what we call 'a low threshold of pain' in some people. How can we find out what causes an excess of naloxene? Could be it 'something we eat'? Many people recognise that pain is closely linked with a lazy, ill-functioning liver (which can also cause mental depression, showing yet again how close are our mental and physical processes).

Studies have shown that patients successfully treated with a placebo experienced a return of pain when given naloxene ('Proceedings of the International Study of Pain 1976', quoted in *Prevention* Vol. 22/6). Brains could be encouraged to fight pain by the use of electrodes but, again, pain relief could be short-circuited if the patient was given a shot of naloxene.

Dr Alex Macdonald, writing in the *General Practitioner* (November 24th 1978) stated that hypnotic analgesia was not inhibited by naloxene. Paul Sacerdote, a psychiatrist who for 25 years had been hypnotising cancer patients to relieve their pain, disagreed.

We could well ask now, how materialist is faith? Perhaps when those therapists who suggest that healing and pain relief depend on what they call 'right thinking' are successful, it is because the patient's ability to believe helps to release the endorphines from the brain without producing too much naloxene at the same time to antidote the analgesic effect. It is surely an obvious field for research. Who knows, someone may discover that small regular doses of smoked salmon (on the NHS of course) are the best way of all to keep naloxene at bay! But if they tell us, will we believe it?

It is sad that just as too many people still think of cancer as a death sentence and incurable, they also imagine hospices are places where the incurably sick go without a return ticket: and essentially religious places at that. No place perhaps for the self-respecting atheist who doesn't believe in or want any Life To Come, who doesn't want to hurt the feelings of those who do, but wants only the opportunity to live to the end with dignity and without religion. Many hospices, however, now make it clear that they do in fact respect the beliefs of patients even if they are non-Christian or non-religious.

Hospices also do their best to inform the public that their specially trained staff pride themselves on welcoming patients in order to control their pain and to see them going home to live lives that are as normal as possible, as often as possible. The work of hospices can be invaluable, but the hospice movement is still tiny in comparison to the need for people to be sure that they will not die alone or in pain.

Whenever the label 'terminal' is used, however, we need to remember how often it is *mis*used by doctors and surgeons. Perhaps there should be a close link forged between groups like Cancer Contact and the hospice movement, so that patients can be sure they will be given the alternative methods of pain control, and a diet that bears no resemblance whatsoever to that in the average hospital. Those of us who are trying to find out how to prevent cancer or restore cancer patients to good health need to be in close touch with those who are primarily concerned with our failures. Cancer Contact is making its own investigations and hoping for just such co-operation.

IV. Cancer Contact Looks Ahead

In 1980 Jill Louw was given a life expectancy of two years. Three years later she and her husband wrote of their cancer experience. Their stories were tragically typical. Jill had refused to have a mastectomy in spite of emotional blackmail, which suggested that she owed it to her family to have the amputation. Her consultant's general comment had been: 'It's a shame that women are learning more about their bodies; it's making my job more difficult.' Jill wrote that although she had now been declared cancer-free, her confidence in a long-term survival had been destroyed.

Ken Louw's story was hardly more encouraging, for the doctor had tried to enlist him, saying patronisingly: 'Women become very emotional over these things.' He supported his wife's decisions but wrote: 'At the time I did not really have anyone I could talk to about it, mainly because I did not have any friends who had had the same experience.'

Cancer Contact had, for more than a year, provided 'someone to talk to', and as a mutually supportive group (with eleven regular members and several more 'homebound') had been successful. Its meetings continued to be lively, constructive, cheerful and comforting. The father of one young member sent a generous donation, and wrote: 'We have just been visiting our daughter, whom we found in great spirits and looking well. It is difficult to properly express the gratitude that absent parents feel towards your group for the support and encouragement and practical help you have given her.' That letter was quite as valuable as the cheque.

The situation of the different members changed all

the time. It was considered 'promotion' to move from being checked every three months to a six-monthly visit to the consultant. But sometimes we were demoted and back to more regular examinations.

The origins of Cancer Contact lay within the Mid-Sussex Homoeopathic Group, but as it grew and developed it began to need its own organisation and funds. Kind neighbours agreed to act as treasurer and fund-raiser, and, if possible, to gather together a group of healthy helpers. Our aims and purposes could be summed up as 'helping people to live with cancer', and so that people could contact us we decided to publicise one telephone number from which enquirers could be given whatever address was appropriate at the time. Each newcomer needed an introductory session with one or two of us to listen and explain what we were trying to do. If they were fit enough (and could arrange transport) they would then join the monthly meetings and make their own friends for further contact.

We already had an interesting collection of relevant books, informative leaflets, as well as two cassette recorders with various tapes on relaxation and visualisation therapy, and we were hoping to arrange for a homoeopathic consultant to answer general questions by this method. We had a bio-feedback machine, 'C' sticks and litmus paper for testing Vitamin C excretion and alkalinity, and there were books, Vitamin C, and Jason Winters' tea for sale. We were relying on donations to pay our running expenses and were grateful for the generosity of all those who helped us.

At our most ambitious and unrealistic we planned a group for the young offspring of cancer patients who needed to talk and ask questions outside their family, with perhaps a young doctor to guide them. We wanted to arrange home visiting for the house-bound and transport for the less-than-mobile. An

Answerphone would be useful, but who was going to deal with the messages? If there were someone to organise public meetings or conferences there need be no shortage of interesting speakers, as we were already getting in touch with anyone we heard was involved with unorthodox cancer research. Gradually, however, we reminded one another of our limitations and agreed that Cancer Contact must stay small or it would fail in its purpose. It wasn't a society of like-minded people trying to enrol members: it was a group of people fighting the same disease and having to find more energy for every newcomer. Sadly we lowered our sights.

We had agreed between us on many points. We were not cancer 'victims'. We had no intention of laying down any laws, only of offering information about as many alternative therapies as possible without any dogmas. No one's beliefs (or lack of faith) were to be criticised. As cancer patients are often seen by others as doomed and in need of swift salvation, we had to make sure that our individual views were respected. We had to learn how to listen with our whole attention, enabling fears, anger or despair to be expressed, while conserving our own energy. Anyone who needed serious counselling should be directed to professionals. We had to avoid getting involved in more than we could comfortably cope with; our own health was our first concern and only when there was energy to spare could we share it with others in need. We were all 'in the same boat' and had the right to say when we were tired, in pain, or just needing a break. All this, in fact, stimulated the idea of 'mutual aid', and people previously overwhelmed with their own miseries found they were now looking after others.

When still part of the MSHG we had begun to send letters out to health visitors, nurses, doctors and anyone who might wish to put cancer patients in touch with us. This letter included the following comments:

> 'We would like you to know what we are trying (and what we shall not be attempting) to do. We accept that cancer is not one but many diseases affecting the whole person. Treatment of local symptoms cannot be enough. No one medical school or system has all the answers, and our health and general well-being are our responsibility. Because it is difficult to kill the cancer without also killing the healthy cells, we have to do everything we can to boost our defence systems so as to try to prevent a further breakdown. We have to find out for ourselves how this can be done according to our own specific idiosyncrasies and needs. And as Lord Acton said: "We must try to understand what we reject as thoroughly as what we accept." We avoid illusions, but we also deplore the negative attitude of those who say that "nothing can be done." Positive thinking is essential.
>
> We want you to know that Cancer Contact will not advise anyone against any treatment prescribed by qualified practitioners.'

It was a decade since one member had met a home-help neighbour who had herself been diagnosed as having 'terminal cancer'. It was exciting that she had been able to announce this loud and clear without any of her previous inhibitions. Talking about cancer had made this possible. The reaction of one friend, however, had been distressing. 'I'm sorry,' she said, 'but if you've got cancer, I'm afraid that is the end of our friendship.' And it was. They never saw each other again. Stories like that were now mercifully thin on the ground but cancerphobia was still liable to appear when least expected. There was also still a steady stream of horror stories emerging from surgeries and hospitals. One GP told her patient: 'God has given you cancer and only God can take it away, but we can arrange meals on wheels for you in due course'! A surgeon who had been a disaster as a communicator repeated his performance by telling the husband of one of our members in four words that his wife was dying, adding: 'I hope you realise it.' Another woman was told that if she went for homoeopathic treatment she need not bother to return to her consultant. She had to find another. And then there was the GP who said to his patient: 'You don't want to go and join a group of other cancer patients sitting around moaning about their problems.' This in fact was more or less just what she did want to do. She joined us — and changed her GP. Most of us had changed our doctors.

We decided that we could probably help cancer patients most if we could get some GPs along to our meetings. And so we sent out invitations. The first agreed that we were a lot of 'fighters' and said he had spent an 'informative evening'. We had to admit that for us it had been a little depressing to hear yet again that apart from orthodox treatment there is little help for the cancer patient, but if we persuaded him that the facts might be otherwise it was an evening well spent.

There can be no blueprint for starting a Cancer Contact group. It all depends on so many things. If you are in the country you may be miles away from a bank or a duplicating machine, but you could find that you are more than compensated by knowing enough people who want to help you. You may, as you can see, have splendid plans but no means of carrying them out, or lots of scope but few ideas.

Some people are of course naturally non-joiners, or want only to be left alone to try to forget they have cancer. Some are quite sure that a collection of cancer patients is bound to be gloomy, morbid, or even paranoid, and only by joining in will they be convinced otherwise. Some people (women especially) are deterred from getting involved because their families don't approve or they feel neglected; we therefore considered the idea of a special group of 'neglected husbands' but that really was impossible to arrange without their co-operation! Cancerphobia is probably at the root of such problems; no one can surely be jealous of a cheerful evening spent by a group of women with cancer! Those spouses who supported us and also what we were trying to do in Cancer Contact were most gratefully appreciated.

There are now many successful self-help groups: CALL (Cancer Aid and Listening Line) in Manchester has an efficient phone-in service, while Mrs Barbara Neale of Eccles-on-Sea (near Norwich) has a fortnightly cancer therapy group for 15-17 people (some of whom travel more than 90 miles to attend) and a monthly group for about 40 people, also in Norwich, concerned with healing and therapy. Some groups of course have no interest in alternative therapies but it is difficult to see how such groups, limited by orthodox attitudes and treatment, can offer a long-term motivation.

We need contacts for cancer patients in every town and village. The medical profession and research scientists have failed miserably to relieve the problems of most cancers. Patients must now help themselves, but if they can help one another with the full co-operation of their medical advisers, so much the better. It was a Dr Ruth Tichauer (the mother of five children) who explained on a TV programme how she works for the Aymara Indians in Bolivia, treating her patients as 'intelligent co-workers in the healing of a case.' Wise woman. Lucky patients.

A Few Tips

The Bristol Cancer Centre suggests a 'cleansing period' of at least two months for 'new' cancer patients. During this time special care should be taken to avoid exhausting the digestion. Here are a few points to remember:

* Cook in steel, enamel, or pyrex; avoid aluminium pans, tea pots, etc. and remember that, if you eat out a

lot, canteen, restaurant (and hospital) kitchens may not be following the same rules.

* Bread. Homemade 100 per cent wholemeal is an ideal basic food containing bran, vitamins, etc. With cane sugar (less than recipes usually say) and dried fruit it makes good cakes if you can't give them up.

* Sweetening. A little honey (honeycomb can help throat problems), dried fruit, or a little cane sugar.

* Salt. Enough only to make food palatable. Horseradish may help to prevent craving.

* Tea. Jason Winters' (from Gerard House, 736 Christchurch Road, Boscombe, Bournemouth, Dorset BH7 6BZ), red clover, and fenugreek tea (recommended by Italian women with breast cancer). Parsley tea an excellent diuretic.

* Coffee. Avoid both real and decaffeinated; try substitutes.

* Raw vegetables and fruit every day, but if they disagree with you not after midday.

* Vegetarians — make sure you balance pulses, beans and grain to get enough proteins. 1 cup of beans to 2⅜ cups of rice is a good balance. Sprout your own seeds and experiment with juices.

* Yoghourt. Home-made is much cheaper than that sold in shops. The sweetened, coloured varieties bear little relation to the real thing, which is supposed to be good for cancer of the colon. A 'must' after antibiotics.

* Grapes and grapejuice are said to have the power to inactivate viruses, and are an excellent source of potassium.

* A clove of garlic every day is another well-tried remedy. Take it first thing, followed by a hot cup of tea and no halitosis! Others swear by almonds eaten daily.

* Diets should be as varied and as enjoyable as possible. When two contradictory diets are recommended for two complaints in the same patient, choose what you like best from each. If you and your family have to eat quite different things, take Dr Bach remedies for frustration and exhaustion.

Glossary

Allopathy The orthodox medical system of treatment: non-homoeopathic.
Adenoma A benign tumour.
Benign Non-malignant: a mild condition which may or may not need treatment.
Biopsy The removal of a small piece of tissue for examination by a pathologist to determine whether or not it is malignant. *Excision biopsy* is the removal of the whole lump.
Carcinogen Any agent believed to cause cancer.
Carcinoma A malignant ('solid') tumour.
Chemotherapy Treatment by one or more anti-cancer (cytoxic) drugs.
Chemotaxis The ability of white blood cells to travel to the site of an injury upon chemical stimulation.
Collagen Gelatinous base of connective tissue.
Colostomy Artificial means of removing the body's waste matter.
Cyst An accumulation of material, usually fluid, in a non-malignant swelling: only very rarely associated with cancer.
Dysplasia Abnormal tissue development.
Epithelial Epithelial cells constitute skin, epidermis and mucous membranes.
Frozen section A small piece of suspect tissue removed during a biopsy, frozen and sent for immediate examination.
Histology Science of organic tissue, hence Histolic Analysis.
Hormone A chemical substance produced in certain parts of the body, which has a specific effect on the activity of one or more distant organs.
Hyperalimentation Artificial feeding with processed proteins, carbohydrates, and fats with minerals and vitamins.

Immunology The study of the way the body defends itself against disease. *Immunosuppressive* refers to any agent which prevents these defence mechanisms from operation. *Immunotherapy* is treatment based on the principle of supporting or improving the body's natural defence mechanisms.
Implant Artificial substance, usually silicone gel, which is inserted into breast cavity to replace the natural breast.
Iatrogenic When illness is produced by treatment.
Iscador Homoeopathically potentised mistletoe used in the treatment of cancer.
Leukemia 'Haematologic neoplasms' — the over-production of leukocytes (white blood cells) which usually cause a marked rise in the number of them circulating in the blood.
Lumpectomy Surgical removal of the lump (tumour), increasingly used as an alternative to mastectomies for breast cancer.
Lymph Colourless fluid from body tissue which resembles blood but has no red corpuscles. *Lymph Gland/Node:* a small mass of tissue where lymph is purified and lymphocytes are formed.
Lymphoma Solid tumours from lymphoid tissue (i.e. lymph nodes and spleen). The most common are Hodgkin's disease and Lymphosarcomas.
Lymphodoema Swelling of arm by fluid which is unable to drain away normally because lymph nodes have been removed.
Malignant In cancer, this refers to growths which are not benign and will spread unless removed or effectively treated.
Mammary gland The breast in women.
Mastectomy Surgical removal of the whole breast.
Metastasis The process by which the malignant cells detach themselves from the primary tumour and establish themselves elsewhere, starting new tumours called 'Metastases' or 'Secondaries'.

Neoplasia Cancer.
Neoplasm Malignant tumour.
Oncology The study of the causes, development, characteristics and treatment of cancer.
Oopherectomy Removal of the ovaries by surgery or radiation.
Orchidectomy Removal of testicles.
Pituitary gland (Also knows as Hypophysis) A small organ at the base of the brain which is responsible for synthesising and releasing at least nine different hormones. Exerts important influence on growth and bodily functions.
Prognosis Medical prediction about the development of disease (often contradicted by others of equal medical calibre).
Prolactin Hormone secreted by the pituitary gland which stimulates the milk flow.
Prophylactic Medical action to prevent disease.
Prosthesis Artificial replacement of part of the anatomy: where there has been a mastectomy, the term applies equally to surgical implants and 'falsies' designed to put into an empty bra.
Radiotherapy Treatment by ionizing radiation: X-rays or cobalt.
Remission A period of good health after the onset of cancer which can happen spontaneously or be the result of effective treatment.
Sarcoma Solid tumour from connective tissue such as cartilage, muscle, fat and bone. Only about 2 per cent of human malignancies are sarcomas, which can be fast-growing.
Steroids Large group of organic compounds which include cholesterol, the sex hormones and the D-vitamins, sometimes used in the treatment of cancer.
Tumour Swelling mass of tissues derived from pre-existing cells which serves no purpose and grows independently of surrounding tissues.

Some Reference Books

1 Wilfred Barlow *The Alexander Principle* (Arrow 1979)
2 Wilfred Barlow (ed.) *More Talk of Alexander* (Gollancz 1978)
3 Margery Blackie *The Challenge of Homoeopathy* (Unwin 1981)
4 Boericks *Materia Medica with Repertory* (Homoeopathic, USA 1927)
5 Victor Bott *Anthroposophical Medicine* (Chapter 14 'The Problem of Cancer' by Dr G. Douch) (Rudolf Steiner Press 1982)
6 Mark Bricklin *Practical Encyclopaedia of Natural Healing* (Rodale, USA 1976)
7 Barbara Brosnan *Yoga for Handicapped People* (Souvenir 1983)
8 Dr Isaac Bryant *Cancer: the Alternative Method of Treatment* (Roberts Publications nd)
9 Maurice Burke *My Successful Fight Against Cancer* (Burke 1982)
10 Fritjof Capra *The Tao of Physics* (Fontana 1978)
11 Mildred Carter *Helping Yourself with Foot Reflexology* (USA 1969)
12 Leon Chaitow *About Laetrile* (Thorsons 1981)
13 Philip M Chancellor *Handbook of Bach Flower Remedies* (C.W. Daniel 1977)
14 Susan E. Charmine *The Complete Raw Juice Therapy* (Thorsons 1981)
15 Arthur Coca, MD *The Pulse Test: Easy Allergy Detection* (Arco, USA 1979)
16 Dr. Vernon Coleman *Bodypower – the Secret of Self Healing* (Thames & Hudson 1983)
17 Stephanie Cook *Second Life* (Michael Joseph 1982)
18 Trevor Cook *Samuel Hahnemann* (Thorsons 1981)
19 A.B. Downing *Euthanasia and the Right to Death: the Case for Voluntary Euthanasia* (Peter Owen 1974)
20 Robert Eagle *Alternative Medicine* (Futura 1978)
21 Dr Hans Ewald *Acupressure Techniques* (Thorsons 1978)

22 Carolyn Faulder *Breast Cancer* (Virago 1982)
23 Dr Maud Tresillian Fere *Does Diet Cure Cancer?* (Thorsons 1971)
24 Max Gerson MD *A Cancer Therapy* (Totality Books, USA 1977)
25 Dr Joan Gomez *A Dictionary of Symptoms* (Paladin 1970)
26 S.J. Haught *Has Dr. Max Gerson a True Cancer Cure?* (Major Books, USA 1979)
27 James Hewitt *Yoga* (Teach Yourself Books 1960)
28 Francis Hitching *Pendulum – the PSI Connection* (Fontana 1977)
29 Brian Inglis *The Disease of Civilisation* (Hodder & Stoughton 1981)
30 Lucien Israel *Conquering Cancer* (Penguin 1980)
31 Don C. Matchan *Reflexology* (Thorsons 1980)
32 Brenda Kidman *A Gentle Way with Cancer* (Century 1982)
33 Alan Klass *There's Gold in Them Thar Pills* (Penguin 1975)
34 Dr A. Leroi *The Cell, the Human Organism and Cancer* (New Knowledge Books nd)
35 Master T.T. Liang *T'ai Chi Ch'uan* (Vintage, USA 1977)
36 Dr Richard Mackarness *Not All in the Mind* (Pan 1978)
37 Eric Maple *Magic, Medicine and Quackery* (Robert Hale 1968)
38 Ainslie Meares MD *The Wealth Within* (Hill of Content, Australia 1982)
39 Arabella Melville and Colin Johnson *Cured to Death* (Secker & Warburg 1982)
40 Earl Mindell *The Vitamin Bible* (Arlington 1979)
41 G. Ruthven Mitchell *Homoeopathy* (W.H. Allen 1975)
42 Kit Mouat *Coping with Cancer* (leaflet 25p from Cancer Contact)
43 H.L. Newbold *Vitamin C Against Cancer* (Stein & Day 1979)

44 Maesimund B. Panos MD and Jane Heimlich *Homoeopathy – Medicine at Home* (Corgi 1982)
45 Dr Peter Parish *Medicines – a Guide for Everybody* (Penguin 1979)
46 Dr Richard Passwater *Cancer and its Nutritional Therapies* (Pivot, USA 1978)
47 Dr Richard Passwater *Evening Primrose Oil (A Good Health Guide)* (Keats, USA 1981)
48 Miriam Polunin *Minerals – What they are and Why we Need them* (Thorsons 1979)
49 John A. Richardson MD and Patricia Griffin RN *Laetrile Case Histories* (USA 1977)
50 Nancy Robinson and Ian Swash *Mastectomy* (Thorsons 1977)
51 Dick Richards MD *Topic of Cancer – When the Killing Has to Stop* (Pergamon 1982)
52 Cyril Scott *Victory over Cancer without Radium or Surgery* (Health Science Press 1971)
53 Cyril Scott *Cancer Prevention* (Athene Publishing Co. 1980)
54 Keith A Scott MB and Lindia McCourt *Homoeopathy* (Thorsons 1980)
55 Paul Simons *Lecithin – the Fat Fighter* (Thorsons 1980)
56 O. Carl Simonton MD, Stephanie Matthews-Simonton, James L. Creighton *Getting Well Again* (Bantam 1981)
57 Carlson Wade *Vitamins & Other Food Supplements and Your Health* (Keats, USA 1974)
58 Nora Weeks *The Medical Discoveries of Edward Bach Physician* (C.W. Daniel 1973)
59 David Widgery *Health in Danger* (Macmillan 1978)
60 Jason Winters *The Jason Winters Story Killing Cancer* (Skilton and Shaw 1980)